Workbook for Providing Home Care A Textbook for Home Health Aides

SEVENTH EDITION

Hartman Publishing, Inc.

hartmanonline.com

Hartman

Credits

Managing Editor
Susan Alvare Hedman

Cover Designer
Kirsten Browne

Cover Illustrator
Iveta Vaicule

Production
Tracy Kopsachilis

Proofreaders
Sapna Desai
Zella Mansson

Copyright Information

1313 Iron Ave SW
Albuquerque, New Mexico 87102
(505) 291-1274
web: hartmanonline.com
email: orders@hartmanpublishing.com

ISBN 978-1-60425-169-2

PRINTED IN THE USA

Notice to Readers

Though the guidelines and procedures contained in this text are based on consultations with healthcare professionals, they should not be considered absolute recommendations. The instructor and readers should follow employer, local, state, and federal guidelines concerning healthcare practices. These guidelines change, and it is the reader's responsibility to be aware of these changes and of the policies and procedures of her or his healthcare facility.

The publisher, author, editors, and reviewers cannot accept any responsibility for errors or omissions or for any consequences from application of the information in this book and make no warranty, express or implied, with respect to the contents of the book. The publisher does not warrant or guarantee any of the products described herein or perform any analysis in connection with any of the product information contained herein.

Gender Usage

This workbook uses gender pronouns interchangeably to denote healthcare team members and clients. The words *male* and *female* as used throughout relate to a person's sex assigned at birth. This may be different from their experienced gender.

Table of Contents

Preface

Welcome to the *Workbook for Providing Home Care: A Textbook for Home Health Aides*! This workbook is designed to help you review what you have learned from reading your textbook. For this reason, the workbook is organized around learning objectives, just like the textbook and your instructor's teaching material.

These learning objectives work as a built-in study guide. After completing the exercises for each learning objective in the workbook, ask yourself if you can DO what that learning objective describes.

If you can, move on to the next learning objective. If you cannot, just go back to the textbook, reread that learning objective, and try again.

We have provided procedure checklists at the end of the workbook. The answers to the workbook exercises are in your instructor's teaching guide.

Happy learning!

1

Home Care and the Healthcare System

1. Describe the structure of the healthcare system and describe ways it is changing

Matching

For each of the following terms, write the letter of the correct definition from the list below. Use each letter only once.

1. ____ Facilities
2. ____ HMOs (health maintenance organizations) and PPOs (preferred provider organizations)
3. ____ Managed care
4. ____ Medicare and Medicaid
5. ____ Payers
6. ____ Providers

(A) Cost-control strategies employed by many health insurance plans

(B) People or organizations that provide health care

(C) Places where health care is delivered or administered

(D) Health insurance plans that seek to control costs by limiting plan members' choice of healthcare providers and facilities

(E) People or organizations paying for health-care services

(F) Forms of public health insurance

Multiple Choice

Circle the letter of the answer that best completes the statement or answers the question.

7. Another name for a long-term care facility is
   (A) Skilled nursing facility
   (B) Home healthcare agency
   (C) Hospital
   (D) Adult day services facility

8. Assisted living facilities are for
   (A) People who need 24-hour skilled care
   (B) People who need some help with daily tasks
   (C) People who will die within 6 months
   (D) People who need acute care

9. Care given by specialists to restore or improve function after an illness or injury is called
   (A) Acute care
   (B) Subacute care
   (C) Rehabilitation
   (D) Hospice care

10. Care given to people who have approximately 6 months or less to live is called
    (A) Acute care
    (B) Subacute care
    (C) Rehabilitation
    (D) Hospice care

2. Explain Medicare and Medicaid, and list when Medicare recipients may receive home care

True or False

Mark each statement with either a T for true or an F for false.

1. ____ To qualify for home health care, Medicare recipients usually must be unable to leave home.
2. ____ Medicare pays for any care that the recipient wants to have.
3. ____ Medicare only covers people aged 65 or older.
4. ____ One reason that a person may qualify for Medicaid is that he has a low income.
5. ____ Home health care is not covered by Medicare.
6. ____ Medicare has two parts: hospital care and doctor services.
7. ____ Medicare pays for 24-hour-a-day home health care.

3. Explain the purpose of and need for home health care

Fill in the Blank

Fill in the blanks with the correct word for each of the following statements.

1. Home care is less ______________________ than a long stay at a hospital or extended care facility.
2. The growing numbers of ______________ people and ____________ ____________ people are also creating a demand for home care services.
3. Healthcare professionals are focused on providing ____________-____________ care.
4. One important reason for home health care is that most people who are ill feel more ______________________ at home.

4. List key events in the history of home care services

Multiple Choice

1. What event happened in 1959 that identified the need for home health care?
   (A) Homemakers were ordered to war so they were unable to help out at home.
   (B) A national conference on homemaker services was held.
   (C) The Medicare program was created.
   (D) A national holiday commemorating homemakers was established.
2. When was Medicare created?
   (A) 1912
   (B) 1996
   (C) 1965
   (D) 1959
3. Why has interest in home health care increased?
   (A) The population of elderly people and people with chronic diseases has grown.
   (B) Many hospitals have closed due to lack of business.
   (C) Healthcare costs have decreased.
   (D) Insurance companies often cover 100% of the costs of home health care.
4. What is the function of a diagnosis-related group (DRG)?
   (A) It pairs people with like illnesses together to form a support system.
   (B) It offers formal training for people with disabilities to reenter the workplace.
   (C) It specifies the treatment cost that Medicare or Medicaid will pay for various diagnoses.
   (D) It provides financial assistance for people with debilitating illnesses.

Name: ______________________________

5. Identify the basic methods of payment for home health services

Short Answer

Answer each of the following in the space provided.

1. Identify five basic methods of payment for home health services.

____

____

____

____

____

2. What happens when an agency's cost of providing care for a client exceeds the Medicare payment?

____

____

____

____

____

6. Describe a typical home health agency

Labeling

Fill in the four blanks below to complete the organizational chart of a typical home health agency. Some sections have already been completed.

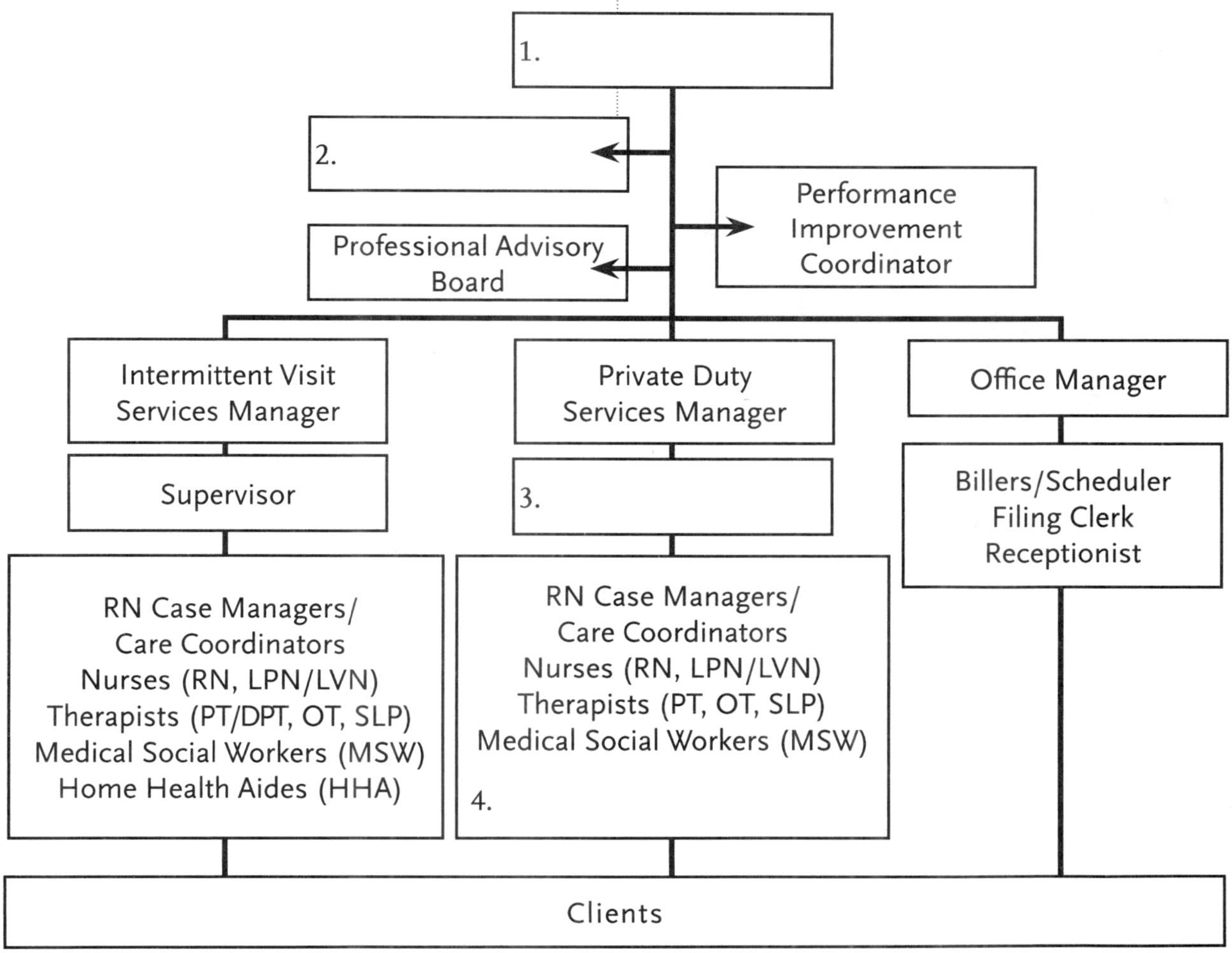

Name: ______________________

7. Explain how working for a home health agency is different from working in other types of facilities

Fill in the Blank

1. A home health aide (HHA) must be aware of personal ______________________ when traveling alone to visit clients.
2. An HHA may have a lot more contact with clients' ______________________ in the home than in a facility.
3. A supervisor monitors an HHA's work, but the most hours will be spent working with clients without direct supervision. Thus, the HHA must be an independent and ______________________ worker.
4. Careful written and verbal ______________________ skills are important.
5. An HHA needs to be ______________________ in order to adapt to changes in the environment.
6. In a client's home, the HHA is a ______________________ and should be respectful of the client's property and customs.

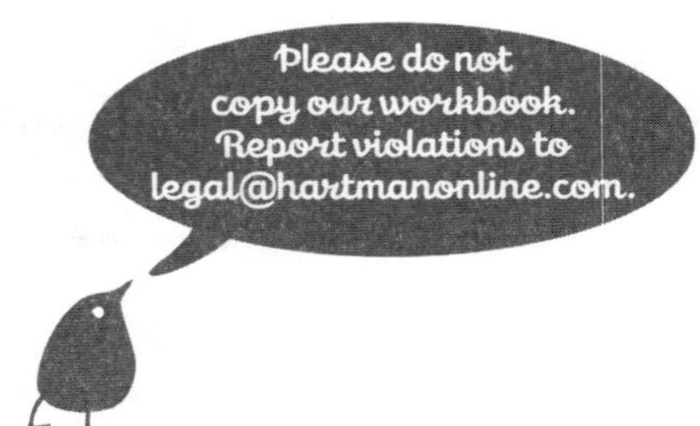

2

The Home Health Aide and the Care Team

1. Identify the role of each care team member

Matching

Use each letter only once.

1. ____ Advanced practice registered nurse (APRN)
2. ____ Case manager or supervisor
3. ____ Client
4. ____ Home health aide (HHA)
5. ____ Medical social worker (MSW)
6. ____ Occupational therapist (OT)
7. ____ Physical therapist (PT or DPT)
8. ____ Physician or doctor (MD or DO)
9. ____ Registered dietitian (RD or RDN)
10. ____ Registered nurse (RN)
11. ____ Speech-language pathologist (SLP)

(A) Develops a treatment plan to improve movement and administers therapy in the form of heat, cold, massage, ultrasound, electrical stimulation, and exercise to muscles, bones, and joints

(B) Coordinates, manages, and provides care, as well as supervises and trains HHAs; develops HHA assignments

(C) Diagnoses disease or disability and prescribes treatment

(D) Creates each client's care plan, monitors changes observed and reported by the HHA, and makes changes to the care plan when necessary

(E) Helps clients get support services, such as counseling and meal services

(F) Performs assigned tasks, such as measuring vital signs, providing personal care, and reporting observations to other care team members

(G) Assesses a client's nutritional status and develops a diet to meet client needs

(H) A registered nurse who has completed training at the postgraduate level (master's or doctoral)

(I) Identifies communication disorders and creates a care plan; teaches exercises to help the client improve or overcome speech impediments

(J) Person whose condition, goals, priorities, treatment, and progress are what the care team revolves around

(K) Helps clients learn to adapt to disabilities by training them to perform activities of daily living, often with the use of assistive devices

2. Describe the role of the home health aide and explain typical tasks performed

Short Answer

1. What are two ways in which home health aides maintain the independence, health, and well-being of clients?

____

____

____

____

Name: ______________________

2. List and give examples of two ways in which home health aides provide services to their clients.

____

____

____

____

____

____

____

____

____

3. Identify tasks outside the scope of practice for home health aides

True or False

1. ____ HHAs do not administer medications unless they are trained and assigned to do so.
2. ____ HHAs can perform invasive procedures.
3. ____ HHAs should ignore any requests that are outside of their scope of practice.
4. ____ HHAs must not accept any request that is not part of their job description or that is not on the assignment sheet.
5. ____ The correct way to deal with an unacceptable request is to explain why the request cannot be met and report it to the supervisor.
6. ____ HHAs do not perform procedures that require sterile technique.
7. ____ It is acceptable for HHAs to prescribe certain medications if they have permission from their supervisor.
8. ____ HHAs should only inform the client or family of a diagnosis or medical treatment plan if the client asks.
9. ____ HHAs may perform any task for which they have been trained, even if it is not part of their assignment.

4. Discuss the client care plan

Complete the Sentence

In each of the following sentences, underline the correct choice between the words or phrases in italics.

1. The client care plan is individualized for each *possible diagnosis* | *client.*
2. Activities not listed on the care plan should *not be performed* | *only be performed if the HHA has extra time.*
3. The care plan includes the client's diagnosis and interventions, such as *medications and treatment* | *hobbies and interests.*

5. Describe how each team member contributes to the care plan

Short Answer

List contributions that each of the following care team members might make in developing the care plan.

1. Home health aide (HHA)

____

____

____

2. Case manager or supervisor

____

____

____

3. Doctor (MD or DO)

____

____

____

4. Medical social worker (MSW)

____

____

____

6. List the federal regulations that apply to home health aides

Multiple Choice

1. HHAs must complete at least ____ hours of training before they begin working in a Medicare-participating agency.
   (A) 30
   (B) 50
   (C) 75
   (D) 100
2. At least how many hours of annual education (in-service training) must HHAs complete?
   (A) 12
   (B) 62
   (C) 75
   (D) 19
3. What is the name of the federal government agency that makes rules to protect workers from bloodborne pathogens and other hazards while on the job?
   (A) Occupational Safety and Health Administration (OSHA)
   (B) Office of the Attorney General (OAG)
   (C) Environmental Protection Agency (EPA)
   (D) Department of Education (DOE)

7. Describe the purpose of the chain of command

Multiple Choice

1. Which of the following statements is true of the chain of command?
   (A) It describes the line of authority.
   (B) It is the same as the care team.
   (C) It details the process for granting medical licenses to home health aides.
   (D) Home health aides are at the top of the chain of command.
2. Liability is a legal term that means
   (A) The line of authority in an agency
   (B) Ignoring a client's request
   (C) Someone can be held responsible for harming someone else
   (D) Not showing up on days that a person is scheduled to work
3. Why should home health aides not do tasks that are not assigned to them?
   (A) The HHA may be assigned more work if he performs additional tasks.
   (B) The HHA may put himself or a client in danger.
   (C) The HHA may need to pay for additional training.
   (D) The HHA may have to arrive at work earlier.
4. What is one reason that licensed healthcare professionals will show great interest in the work that an HHA does?
   (A) They may not trust the HHA.
   (B) They assign tasks to the HHA.
   (C) They may not have much respect for the HHA.
   (D) They can avoid having to pay the HHA if she makes a mistake.

8. Define *policies* and *procedures* and explain why they are important

Short Answer

List five examples of common policies and procedures at home health agencies.

1. ______________________

____

____

2. ______________________

____

____

3. ______________________

____

____

Name: ______________________

4. ______________________

5. ______________________

9. List examples of a professional relationship with a client and an employer

Short Answer

Read each of the following scenarios and answer the questions.

1. Kathy, an HHA, wakes up late and decides to skip her morning shower to make up for lost time. She also skips breakfast because she wants to make her first assignment on time. Because she is feeling so rushed, she forgets to respond when her client says, "Good morning." Instead, she complains to her client about her sleepless night, headache, and lack of breakfast.

   How could Kathy have behaved more professionally?

   ____

2. At her next client's home, Kathy asks to use the bathroom. She washes her hands carefully when she is finished and begins to prepare her client's lunch. She listens to her client talk about his grandchildren's visit the day before and encourages her client to share photographs of the grandchildren. As Kathy is leaving, her client offers her a gift. Kathy politely refuses the gift and explains that it is against her agency's policy.

   List all the examples of Kathy's professional behavior.

   ____

3. Cornel, an HHA, runs out of time at one client's home and is unable to finish his assignment. When his supervisor finds out, she tells him that he needs to work more efficiently. This makes Cornel very upset, and he begins to wonder if his job is worth all the criticism he seems to be getting.

   How could Cornel respond more professionally?

   ____

4. At his next meeting with his supervisor, Cornel explains why he was unable to finish his assignment and asks his supervisor for suggestions. She shows him how to organize his time more efficiently. After asking several more questions, Cornel feels that he understands how to work more effectively. Being able to communicate in a positive way with his supervisor improves Cornel's attitude about his job.

   List all the examples of Cornel's professional behavior.

   ____

____

____

____

10. Demonstrate how to organize care assignments

Short Answer

1. Why is it important for an HHA to organize their work?

____

____

____

____

____

____

____

2. Why should the HHA include the client in planning his schedule?

____

____

____

____

____

____

____

11. Demonstrate proper personal grooming habits

Multiple Choice

1. Which of these products should an HHA use every day?
   (A) Makeup to cover blemishes
   (B) Deodorant
   (C) Body spray
   (D) Scented lotion

2. Which of the following should an HHA wear to work?
   (A) Dangling earrings
   (B) An identification badge
   (C) Aftershave lotion
   (D) Acrylic nails

3. Proper grooming for an HHA includes
   (A) Hair that is tied back if it is long
   (B) Long, trimmed beards
   (C) Long, clean nails
   (D) Dramatic eye makeup

4. Which shoes would be the best choice for an HHA to wear to work?
   (A) Supportive athletic shoes
   (B) Slip-on shoes with an open back
   (C) Soft, cushioned sandals
   (D) Polished dress shoes

12. Identify personal qualities a home health aide must have

Matching

Use each letter only once.

1. _____ Compassionate
2. _____ Conscientious
3. _____ Dependable
4. _____ Empathetic
5. _____ Honest
6. _____ Organized
7. _____ Patient
8. _____ Proactive
9. _____ Respectful
10. _____ Sympathetic
11. _____ Tactful
12. _____ Unprejudiced

(A) Being caring, concerned, considerate, empathetic, and understanding

(B) Giving the same quality of care, regardless of age, gender, sexual orientation, gender identity, religion, race, ethnicity, body size, or condition

(C) Guided by a sense of right and wrong

(D) Valuing other people's individuality and treating others politely and kindly

(E) Speaking and acting without offending others

(F) Being able to manage time well, plan ahead, and prioritize tasks

(G) Being truthful

(H) Getting to work on time and doing assigned tasks skillfully

(I) Anticipating potential problems and needs before they occur

(J) Identifying with the feelings of others

(K) Sharing in the feelings and difficulties of others

(L) Not losing one's temper easily; not acting irritated or annoyed; not rushing clients

13. Identify an employer's responsibilities

Short Answer

List and describe seven responsibilities of the employer to the HHA.

1. ______

2. ______

3. ______

4. ______

5. ______

6. ______

7. ______

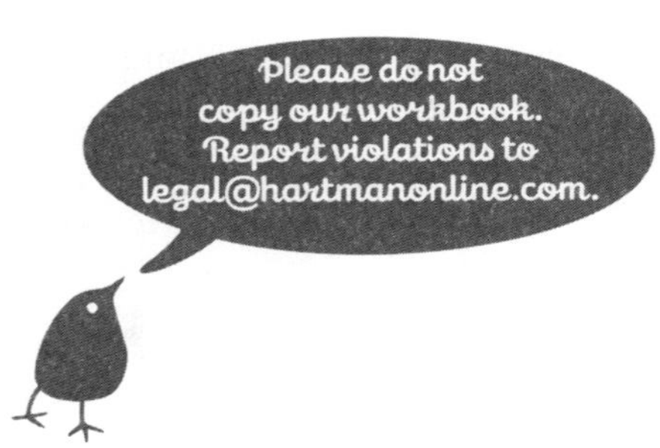

3

Legal and Ethical Issues

1. Define the terms *ethics* and *laws* and list examples of legal and ethical behavior

Short Answer

1. Sarah, an HHA, is out shopping with her friends. One of them asks her if she likes her job, and she responds enthusiastically. She proceeds to tell them that her client, Mrs. Hernandez, has Alzheimer disease and has to be reminded of her name several times a day, as she is apt to forget it.

   Did Sarah behave in a legal and ethical manner? Why or why not?

   ____

   ____

   ____

   ____

   ____

   ____

2. Caroyl, an HHA, finishes her duties for the day early. Her client, Mr. Kim, tells her how pleased he is with her work. He says that she is the first aide that has made him feel so comfortable and well taken care of. He gives her a little box of candy and says it is for all the hard work she has done. Caroyl initially refuses, but after he insists, she takes it from him, thanking him.

   Did Caroyl behave in a legal and ethical manner? Why or why not?

   ____

   ____

   ____

   ____

   ____

   ____

3. Mark, an HHA, has been working for Mrs. Stein for almost a year. Her family is visiting from out of state and Mark meets her daughter, Susan, for the first time. During the course of conversation, Susan asks Mark to come have a drink with her so that they can talk about her mother's case in a more relaxed environment. Mark tells her that he can go out for a short while. They arrange to meet.

   Did Mark behave in a legal and ethical manner? Why or why not?

   ____

   ____

   ____

   ____

   ____

   ____

2. Explain clients' rights and discuss why they are important

True or False

1. ____ If an HHA knows that a client is being abused by a family member, he should immediately confront the abuser.

2. ____ If an HHA suspects that a client is being abused, he should not report it until he has proof that the abuse is actually happening.

3. ____ Clients have the right to participate in their care planning.

4. ____ Clients should only be informed of barriers to their care if they are life-threatening.

5. ____ Neglect is the failure to provide needed care that results in physical, mental, or emotional harm to a person.

6. ____ Clients do not need to know what services they are being charged for, as long as they are receiving adequate care.

Matching

Use each letter only once.

7. ____ Abuse
8. ____ Assault
9. ____ Battery
10. ____ Domestic violence
11. ____ False imprisonment
12. ____ Financial abuse
13. ____ Involuntary seclusion
14. ____ Malpractice
15. ____ Neglect
16. ____ Negligence
17. ____ Physical abuse
18. ____ Psychological abuse
19. ____ Sexual abuse
20. ____ Sexual harassment
21. ____ Substance use disorder
22. ____ Verbal abuse
23. ____ Workplace violence

(A) Actions, or the failure to act or provide the proper care, resulting in unintended injury

(B) The repeated use of legal or illegal substances in a way that harms oneself or others

(C) Any unwelcome sexual advance or behavior that creates an intimidating, hostile, or offensive working environment

(D) The separation of a person from others against the person's will

(E) The unlawful restraint of someone that affects the person's freedom of movement

(F) Verbal, physical, or sexual abuse of staff by other staff members or clients, or clients' family or friends

(G) Intentionally touching a person without permission

(H) The use of words or actions to cause another person to feel fearful of being harmed

(I) The improper or illegal use of a person's money, possessions, property, or other assets

(J) Nonconsensual sexual contact of any type

(K) The use of spoken or written words, pictures, or gestures that threaten, embarrass, or insult a person

(L) Emotional harm caused by threatening, scaring, humiliating, intimidating, isolating, or insulting a person, or by treating an adult like a child

(M) Physical, sexual, or emotional abuse by spouses, intimate partners, or family members

(N) Purposeful mistreatment that causes physical, mental, or emotional pain or injury to someone

(O) Any treatment, intentional or unintentional, that causes harm to a person's body—includes slapping, bruising, cutting, burning, physically restraining, pushing, shoving, and rough handling

(P) Injury caused by professional misconduct through negligence, carelessness, or lack of skill

(Q) Failure to provide needed care that results in physical, mental, or emotional harm to a person

3. List ways to recognize and report elder abuse and neglect

Short Answer

1. Name 10 suspicious injuries that should be reported.

____

____

____

____

____

____

____

____

____

____

____

2. What is a mandated reporter?

____

____

____

____

____

____

4. List examples of behavior supporting and promoting clients' rights

Multiple Choice

1. When performing a procedure on a client, the HHA should
   (A) Try to distract the client so he will not know what the HHA is doing
   (B) Explain the procedure fully before performing it
   (C) Wait until the client is reading before starting the procedure
   (D) Notify the physician first

2. Which of the following would be the best response by an HHA if a client refuses to take a bath?
   (A) The HHA should offer the client a prize if she will take the bath.
   (B) The HHA should respect the client's wishes, but report the refusal to the supervisor.
   (C) The HHA should explain that he might lose his job if the client does not take the bath.
   (D) The HHA should explain to the client why it is wrong not to bathe.

3. An HHA's husband asks her to tell him some personal details about one of her clients. The best response by the HHA would be to
   (A) Explain that she cannot talk about the client
   (B) Tell him a story if he promises to keep it confidential
   (C) Make up a story to tell, so as not to share anything private
   (D) Tell him something that the HHA knows that the client would not mind her sharing

4. If an HHA suspects his client is being abused, he should
   (A) Open the client's mail and look through his belongings to find any clues
   (B) Keep watching the client to make sure his suspicions are correct
   (C) Report it to his supervisor immediately
   (D) Check with other HHAs to get some advice

5. Explain HIPAA and list ways to protect clients' confidentiality

Multiple Choice

1. What is the purpose of HIPAA?
   (A) To monitor quality of care in clients' homes
   (B) To protect and secure the privacy of health information
   (C) To reduce incidents of abuse
   (D) To provide health insurance for uninsured elderly people

2. What is included under protected health information (PHI)?
   (A) Patient's favorite food
   (B) Patient's favorite color
   (C) Patient's social security number
   (D) Patient's library card number

3. What is the correct response by an HHA if someone who is not directly involved with a client's care asks for a client's PHI?
   (A) Give them the information
   (B) Ask the client if they may have the information
   (C) Ask them to send a written request for the information
   (D) Tell them that the information is confidential and cannot be shared

4. Which of the following is one way to keep PHI confidential?
   (A) Making comments about clients on Instagram
   (B) Discussing a client's progress with a coworker in a restaurant
   (C) Not leaving detailed information for clients in voicemail messages
   (D) Only discussing clients' conditions with friends or family members

5. The abbreviation for a law that was enacted as a part of the American Recovery and Reinvestment Act of 2009 to expand the protection and security of consumers' electronic health records is
   (A) HISEAL
   (B) HITECH
   (C) HIHELP
   (D) HIQUIET

6. Discuss and give examples of advance directives

Matching

1. ____ Advance directives
2. ____ Do not hospitalize (DNH) order
3. ____ Do not intubate (DNI) order
4. ____ Do not resuscitate (DNR) order
5. ____ Durable power of attorney for health care
6. ____ Living will
7. ____ Physician Orders for Life-Sustaining Treatment (POLST)

(A) A signed, dated, and witnessed legal document that appoints someone else to make the medical decisions for a person in the event that he becomes unable to do so

(B) Outlines the medical care a person wants, or does not want, in case the person becomes unable to make those decisions; *directive to physicians* and *medical directive* are other terms used to describe this

(C) A medical order that means the person does not want to be sent to the hospital for treatment

(D) Legal documents that allow people to decide what kind of medical care they wish to have if they are unable to make those decisions themselves

(E) A medical order that tells medical professionals not to perform cardiopulmonary resuscitation (CPR)

(F) A medical order that means no breathing tube will be placed in the person, even if some CPR measures are used

(G) A medical order that specifies the treatments a person wants to receive when the person is very ill

7. Identify community resources available to help the elderly

Short Answer

What is one way an HHA can locate community resources for the elderly?

____

____

____

____

4

Communication and Diversity

1. Define communication

Short Answer

1. List the three basic steps of communication.

2. Why is feedback an important part of communication?

3. Why is effective communication a critical part of an HHA's job?

2. Explain verbal and nonverbal communication

Multiple Choice

1. Which of the following is an example of nonverbal communication?
   (A) Asking for a glass of water
   (B) Pointing to a glass of water
   (C) Screaming for a glass of water
   (D) Saying, "I do not like water"

2. Verbal communication includes
   (A) Facial expressions
   (B) Nodding one's head
   (C) Speaking
   (D) Shrugging one's shoulders

3. Types of nonverbal communication include
   (A) Speaking
   (B) Facial expressions
   (C) Yelling
   (D) Oral reports

Name: ______________________

4. Which of the following is an example of a confusing or conflicting message (saying one thing and meaning another)?
   (A) Mr. Williams smiles and tells his HHA that he is excited because his daughter is coming to visit.
   (B) Mr. Sanchez looks like he is in pain. When his HHA asks him about it, Mr. Sanchez tells her that his back has been bothering him.
   (C) Mr. Sanders agrees with his HHA when she says it is a nice day, but Mr. Sanders looks angry.
   (D) Mr. Lee will not watch his favorite TV show. He says he is a little depressed.

5. In the previous question, how could the HHA clarify the confusing or conflicting message?
   (A) State what the HHA has observed and ask if the observation is correct
   (B) Ignore the conflicting message and accept what the client said
   (C) Ask the client to repeat what he just said
   (D) Tell the client that the HHA knows he is not telling the truth

6. Which of the following is true?
   (A) All cultural groups view standing close to another person as a potential threat.
   (B) The use of touch is the same for all cultures.
   (C) Different cultures may have different behaviors, attitudes, and customs.
   (D) Maintaining eye contact while talking is preferred by all cultures.

3. Describe therapeutic communication and identify barriers to communication

Multiple Choice

1. One way for an HHA to be a good listener is to
   (A) Finish a client's sentences for him to show that the HHA understands what the client is saying
   (B) Pretend that the HHA understands what a client is saying even if she does not
   (C) Restate the message in the HHA's own words
   (D) Fill in any pauses to avoid awkwardness

2. Active listening involves
   (A) Focusing on the sender and giving feedback
   (B) Avoiding speaking to the client if the HHA cannot understand him
   (C) Deciding what the client is going to say before he says it
   (D) Talking about the HHA's personal problems to relate to the client

3. Mrs. Velasco is a new client who recently moved to the United States. She speaks English, but sometimes seems uncertain or anxious about communicating with her HHA. What can her HHA do to make her more comfortable?
   (A) Give her advice about how to fit in better with American culture
   (B) Talk constantly so that she will not have to speak
   (C) Learn some words and expressions in her language and communicate with empathy
   (D) Avoid speaking to her while giving care

4. When clients report symptoms or feelings, the best response by the HHA is to
   (A) Give medical advice
   (B) Suggest medications
   (C) Avoid speaking
   (D) Ask for more information

5. Which of the following statements describes a way for an HHA to have positive relationships with clients?
   (A) The HHA should fold her arms in front of her while clients are talking.
   (B) The HHA should tell clients she knows exactly how they feel, so clients will feel that they have something in common.
   (C) The HHA should ignore a client's request if she knows she cannot fulfill it.
   (D) The HHA should try to understand what clients are going through.

6. Mr. Vernon is an elderly client who has terminal cancer. He is telling Katie, his HHA, that he is very depressed about dying. He feels he has left many things unfinished. Hearing this makes Katie uncomfortable. Which of the following would be the best response by Katie?
   (A) She should ignore what he is saying.
   (B) She should try to interest him in a brighter subject.
   (C) She should listen to him and ask questions when appropriate.
   (D) She should tell him she knows exactly how he feels.

7. Which of the following is true of therapeutic communication?
   (A) It includes the HHA learning a new language.
   (B) It involves building trust between a client and HHA.
   (C) It is the same as psychotherapy.
   (D) It only involves communication between the HHA and the rest of the care team.

Crossword

Across

10. Type of terminology that may not be understood by clients or their families; HHAs should speak in simple, everyday words

12. Type of questions that should be asked because they need more than a "yes" or "no" answer

14. Phrases used over and over again that do not really mean anything

Down

8. Type of language that is part of nonverbal communication; HHAs should be aware of this when speaking

9. Being this way and taking time to listen when clients are difficult to understand help promote better communication

11. HHAs cannot offer opinions or give this because it is not within their scope of practice

13. Type of question that should be avoided, as it often makes people feel defensive

15. Type of words and expressions that should not be used by HHAs because they are unprofessional and may not be understood

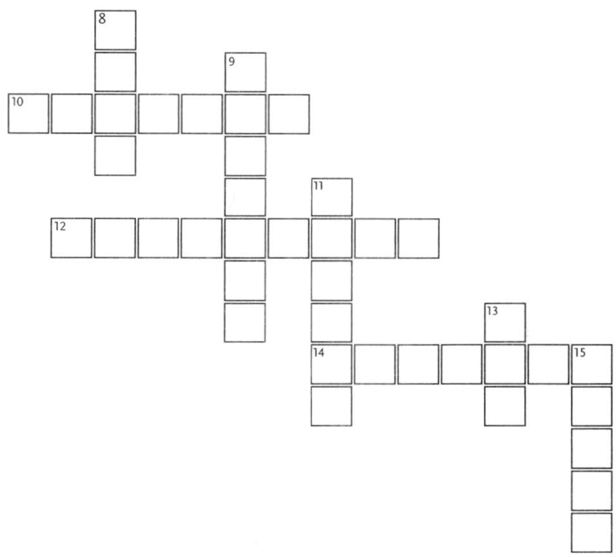

4. Describe the difference between facts and opinions

Short Answer

For each statement made by the HHA, decide whether it is an example of a fact or an opinion. Write F *for fact or* O *for opinion in the space provided.*

1. ____ It is better to take your bath before you eat.

2. ____ You will get depressed if you stay in your pajamas all day.

3. ____ Mr. Ellington sounds angry.

4. ____ My agency says I cannot accept a gift.
5. ____ Your care plan calls for snacks between meals.
6. ____ Ms. Porter did not drink any of her milk at dinner.
7. ____ I think Mr. Holling is lonely.
8. ____ Mr. Larking's pulse was elevated last night after dinner, but it was back to normal this morning.
9. ____ Mr. Ford drinks more coffee than is good for him.
10. ____ Mr. Ford drinks three cups of coffee every morning.
11. ____ Mrs. Myers needs assistance to stand up.
12. ____ Mrs. Myers looks like she is in a lot of pain.

5. Describe basic medical terminology and approved abbreviations

Matching

For each of the following abbreviations, write the letter of the correct term from the list below.

1. ____ ac, a.c.
2. ____ amb
3. ____ BM
4. ____ C
5. ____ c/o
6. ____ CPR
7. ____ F
8. ____ FBS
9. ____ f/u, F/U
10. ____ GI
11. ____ I&O
12. ____ NPO
13. ____ OOB
14. ____ PC, p.c.
15. ____ PRN
16. ____ PWB
17. ____ ROM
18. ____ SOB
19. ____ TPR
20. ____ VS

(A) Fahrenheit degree
(B) Gastrointestinal
(C) After meals
(D) Nothing by mouth
(E) Bowel movement
(F) Cardiopulmonary resuscitation
(G) Complains of
(H) Range of motion
(I) Partial weight-bearing
(J) Temperature, pulse, respirations
(K) Shortness of breath
(L) Before meals
(M) Fasting blood sugar
(N) Vital signs
(O) As necessary
(P) Intake and output
(Q) Celsius degree
(R) Out of bed
(S) Follow-up
(T) Ambulate, ambulatory

6. Explain how to give and receive an accurate oral report of a client's status

Multiple Choice

1. Which of the following is true of oral reports?
   (A) HHAs should use facts when making oral reports.
   (B) HHAs should use opinions when making oral reports.
   (C) HHAs should make oral reports directly to clients' families.
   (D) HHAs do not make oral reports.

2. Which of the following should be reported to the supervisor immediately?
   (A) The client says she had trouble sleeping.
   (B) The client fell.
   (C) The client's family visited.
   (D) The client requested help getting to the toilet.

3. What is the best way for an HHA to remember important details for an oral report?
   (A) Rely on his memory
   (B) Repeat the information to a friend
   (C) Write notes and use them for his report
   (D) Tell another HHA to remind him

7. Explain objective and subjective information and describe how to observe and report accurately

Short Answer

Looking at the diagram, list examples of observations using each sense.

For each of the following, decide whether it is an objective observation (you can see, hear, smell, or touch it) or a subjective observation (the client must tell you about it). Write O for objective and S for subjective.

1. ____ Skin rash
2. ____ Crying
3. ____ Rapid pulse
4. ____ Headache
5. ____ Nausea
6. ____ Vomiting
7. ____ Swelling
8. ____ Cloudy urine
9. ____ Feeling sad
10. ____ Red area on the skin
11. ____ Fever
12. ____ Dizziness
13. ____ Wheezing
14. ____ Chest pain
15. ____ Toothache
16. ____ Coughing
17. ____ Fruity breath
18. ____ Itchy arm

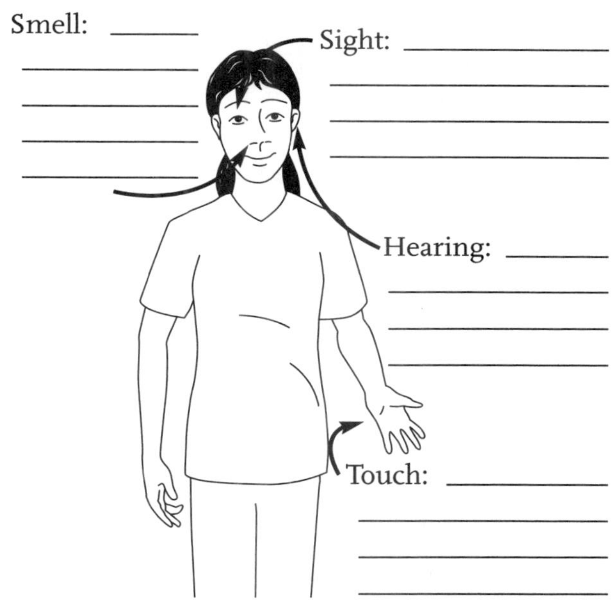

Name: ____________________

8. Explain why documentation is important and describe how to document visit records and incident reports

Multiple Choice

1. Which of the following statements is true of a client's medical chart?
   (A) A medical chart is the legal record of a client's care.
   (B) Not all care needs to be documented.
   (C) The information in a medical chart can be shared with anyone who asks to review it.
   (D) Medical charts are not legal documents.

2. When should care be documented?
   (A) Before care is given
   (B) Immediately after care is given
   (C) At the end of the next day
   (D) Whenever there is time

3. An incident is
   (A) An accident or unexpected event that occurs during a visit
   (B) Any interaction between clients and HHAs
   (C) A normal part of personal care routines
   (D) Any event in a client's day

4. Which of the following would be considered an incident?
   (A) A client complains of a headache.
   (B) A client falls but is fine afterward.
   (C) A client wants his meal brought to his bedroom.
   (D) A client needs to be transferred from his bed to a chair.

5. Which of the following is true of an electronic medical record (EMR)?
   (A) It can be accessed electronically by a single healthcare facility.
   (B) It requires handwritten documentation.
   (C) It can be accessed electronically by many different healthcare facilities and systems.
   (D) HIPAA guidelines do not apply to an EMR.

Short Answer

Convert the following times to military time.

6. 2:10 p.m. ____________________
7. 4:30 a.m. ____________________
8. 10:00 a.m. ____________________
9. 8:25 p.m. ____________________

Convert the following times to regular time.

10. 0600 ____________________
11. 2320 ____________________
12. 1927 ____________________
13. 1800 ____________________

9. Demonstrate the ability to use verbal and written information to assist with the care plan

Short Answer

1. If an HHA is not sure what is important to mention in a care plan meeting, what should he do?

____
____
____
____
____

2. Why is accurate reporting by an HHA so important to the other members of the care team?

____
____
____
____
____

10. Demonstrate effective communication on the telephone

Short Answer

Read the HHA's side of the following telephone conversations and think about how the HHA could have better presented herself on the phone.

Example #1: Leaving a message for the supervisor

Hi, who's this?

Could you get Ms. Crier, please? I need to talk to her.

She's not there? Do you know where she is? I really have to talk to her right now. My client forgot to take her pill this morning, and now she wants to take two. I don't know if that's okay or not, so that's why I need to talk to Ms. Crier.

Okay, well tell her Ella called and have her call me back. Ella. Ella Ferguson. I should be on the schedule.

I don't know how much longer I'll be here, but have her call me as soon as possible. Bye.

1. What did the HHA do incorrectly in this phone conversation?

Example #2: Answering calls for the client

Hello? Mrs. Lee? No, she can't come to the phone right now. She's in the bathroom. Who's calling?

And your number?

Can I tell her what this is about?

Okay. I'll give her the message. Goodbye.

2. What did the HHA do incorrectly in this phone conversation?

11. Discuss diversity and describe common religions

Short Answer

1. What is bias?

2. What are eight types of diversity HHAs may encounter among clients?

Name: ______________________

____

____

____

____

3. Give an example of how a person may be influenced by many different cultures.

____

____

____

____

Matching

Write the letter of the correct description beside each term related to the religious faith or belief. Use each letter only once.

4. ____ Agnosticism
5. ____ Atheism
6. ____ Buddhism
7. ____ Christianity
8. ____ Hinduism
9. ____ Islam
10. ____ Judaism

(A) Praying five times a day facing Mecca and worshipping at mosques are part of this religion's practices.

(B) Being baptized and receiving communion may be part of this religion's practices.

(C) Believing that one does not know or cannot know if God exists

(D) Emphasizing meditation and believing that Nirvana is the highest spiritual plane a person can reach are part of this religion.

(E) Believing in karma is a part of this religion.

(F) Believing that God gave laws through Moses in the form of the Torah is part of this religion.

(G) Actively denying the existence of any deity or higher power

12. List examples of cultural and religious differences

Short Answer

List three examples of dietary restrictions that may be due to religious beliefs.

1. ______________________

____

____

2. ______________________

____

____

3. ______________________

____

____

Multiple Choice

4. Which of the following is the name of a type of diet in which no animals or animal products are consumed, and animal products may not be used or worn?
   (A) Fast
   (B) Vegan
   (C) Kosher
   (D) Lacto-ovo vegetarian

5. Not eating food or eating very little food for a period of time is called
   (A) Bingeing
   (B) Restricting
   (C) Fasting
   (D) Testing

13. List ways of coping with combative behavior

Fill in the Blank

1. ______________________ behavior means being violent or hostile.

2. This behavior may be the result of ______________________________ affecting the brain, an expression of ______________________________, or part of someone's ______________________________.

3. HHAs should try not to take combative behavior ______________________________.

4. HHAs should always ______________________________ and ______________________________ combative behavior.

5. It is important for the care team to be ______________________________ of this behavior, even if the HHA does not find it upsetting.

14. List ways of coping with inappropriate behavior

Short Answer

1. List three examples of client behavior that would be considered inappropriate.

____

____

____

____

____

____

____

____

____

____

____

____

____

____

____

____

____

____

____

2. For each example listed in question 1, describe how an HHA should respond.

____

____

____

____

____

____

____

____

____

____

____

____

____

____

____

____

Name: ______________________________

5

Infection Prevention and Standard Precautions

1. Define *infection prevention* and explain the chain of infection

Multiple Choice

1. The following are necessary links in the chain of infection. Which link is broken by wearing gloves, thus preventing the spread of disease?
   (A) Reservoir (place where the pathogen lives and grows)
   (B) Mode of transmission (a way for the disease to spread)
   (C) Susceptible host (person who is likely to get the disease)
   (D) Portal of exit (body opening that allows pathogens to leave)

2. The following are necessary links in the chain of infection. By getting a vaccination shot for hepatitis B, which link will a person affect to prevent him from getting this disease?
   (A) Reservoir (place where the pathogen lives and grows)
   (B) Mode of transmission (a way for the disease to spread)
   (C) Susceptible host (person who is likely to get the disease)
   (D) Portal of exit (body opening that allows pathogens to leave)

3. The most important thing an HHA can do to prevent the spread of disease is to
   (A) Carry dirty linen close to her uniform
   (B) Put a cap on needles before discarding them
   (C) Remove gloves before cleaning spills
   (D) Wash her hands

4. In what type of environment do microorganisms grow best?
   (A) In a warm, moist place
   (B) In a bright place
   (C) In a cool, dry place
   (D) In a frozen place

2. Explain Standard Precautions

Multiple Choice

1. Standard Precautions should be practiced
   (A) Only on clients who look like they have a bloodborne disease
   (B) On every single client under an HHA's care
   (C) Only on clients who request that the HHA follow them
   (D) Only on clients who have tuberculosis

2. Standard Precautions include the following measures:
   (A) Washing hands after taking off gloves but not before putting on gloves
   (B) Wearing gloves if there is a possibility of coming into contact with blood, body fluids, mucous membranes, or broken skin
   (C) Touching body fluids with bare hands
   (D) Recapping used needles before putting them in the waste container

3. Which of the following is true of Transmission-Based Precautions?
   (A) An HHA does not need to practice Standard Precautions if he practices Transmission-Based Precautions.
   (B) They are exactly the same as Standard Precautions.
   (C) They are practiced in addition to Standard Precautions.
   (D) They are never practiced at the same time that Standard Precautions are used.

4. How should sharps such as needles be disposed of?
   (A) Sharps should be placed in blue recycling containers.
   (B) Sharps should be placed in kitchen trash containers.
   (C) Sharps should be placed inside used gloves and then put in the outside trash receptacle.
   (D) Sharps should be placed in puncture-resistant biohazard containers.

3. Define *hand hygiene* and identify when to wash hands

Multiple Choice

1. An HHA will come into contact with microorganisms
   (A) Only in bathrooms in a house
   (B) Only during direct contact with clients
   (C) Only during personal care procedures
   (D) Every time the HHA touches something

2. The CDC (Centers for Disease Control and Prevention) defines hand hygiene as
   (A) Handwashing with soap and water or using alcohol-based hand sanitizer
   (B) Using only alcohol-based hand rubs
   (C) Rinsing hands with cold water
   (D) Not washing hands more than once per day

3. How long should an HHA use friction when lathering and washing her hands?
   (A) 2 minutes
   (B) 5 seconds
   (C) 18 seconds
   (D) 20 seconds

4. Identify when to use personal protective equipment (PPE)

Short Answer

Make a check mark (✓) next to the tasks that require an HHA to wear gloves.

1. ____ Contact with body fluids
2. ____ Hanging clean laundry
3. ____ When the HHA may touch blood
4. ____ Brushing a client's hair
5. ____ Assisting with perineal care
6. ____ Washing vegetables
7. ____ Giving a massage to a client who has acne on his back
8. ____ Assisting with mouth care
9. ____ Shaving a client

Multiple Choice

10. What type of PPE may be needed when caring for a client with a respiratory illness?
    (A) Eyeglasses and mask
    (B) Mask and foot covering
    (C) Eyeglasses and gloves
    (D) Mask or respirator

11. What type of PPE is used most often by healthcare workers?
    (A) Gloves
    (B) Mask
    (C) Face shield
    (D) Goggles

12. How many times can a gown be worn before it needs to be discarded?
    (A) One time
    (B) Two times
    (C) Three times
    (D) Four times

13. If blood or other body fluids may be splashed or sprayed into the eye area, this PPE can protect the eyes:
    (A) Gloves
    (B) Mask
    (C) Gown
    (D) Goggles

Short Answer

14. What is the correct order for donning (putting on) PPE?

1. ______________________________
2. ______________________________
3. ______________________________
4. ______________________________
5. ______________________________

15. What is the correct order for doffing (removing) PPE?

1. ______________________________
2. ______________________________
3. ______________________________
4. ______________________________
5. ______________________________

5. Explain how to handle spills

Short Answer

Read the following scenario and answer the questions below.

Ritchie, an HHA, collects a urine sample from his client, Mrs. Velasquez. When he finishes, he accidentally knocks the container onto the linoleum floor. Some of the urine spills onto the floor. Ritchie quickly grabs a sponge and begins to wipe up the spill. When he is finished, he finds the mop, puts dishwashing soap into a bucket, and cleans the area again. When he is done mopping, he washes his hands.

Did Ritchie follow the proper spill-handling procedure? If not, what should Ritchie have done?

____

____

____

____

____

____

____

____

____

____

____

6. Explain Transmission-Based Precautions

Short Answer

List the type of precaution being described in each phrase below. Use an A for Airborne Precautions, a C for Contact Precautions, and a D for Droplet Precautions. Each letter may be used more than once.

1. ____ Transmission can occur when touching a contaminated area on the client's body.
2. ____ Used when there is a risk of spreading an infection by direct contact with a person or an object
3. ____ Used to guard against tuberculosis
4. ____ Covering the nose and mouth with a tissue when a person sneezes or coughs, and washing hands immediately after sneezing are part of these precautions.
5. ____ Helps prevent the spread of *Clostridioides difficile* (*C. diff*) and conjunctivitis (pink eye)
6. ____ Used when the microorganisms are spread by droplets in the air that travel only short distances (normally not more than 6 feet)
7. ____ Microorganisms can be spread by coughing, sneezing, talking, or laughing.
8. ____ Helps prevent the spread of pathogens that can float in the air
9. ____ Helps protect against transmission of influenza
10. ____ May require the use of a special mask, such as an N95 or HEPA respirator

7. Explain sterilization and disinfection

Short Answer

1. How would an HHA use wet heat to disinfect? How would an HHA use dry heat to disinfect?

____

____

____

____

____

____

2. What is the difference between sterilization and disinfection?

____

____

____

____

____

____

8. Explain how bloodborne diseases are transmitted

Multiple Choice

1. Bloodborne diseases can be transmitted by
   (A) Infected blood entering the bloodstream
   (B) Hugging a person with a bloodborne disease
   (C) Being in the same room as a person with a bloodborne disease
   (D) Talking to a person with a bloodborne disease

2. In health care, the most common way to be infected with a bloodborne disease is by
   (A) Contact with infected blood or other body fluids
   (B) Hugging a client with a bloodborne disease
   (C) Being in the same room as a client with a bloodborne disease
   (D) Touching tissues used by an infected client

9. Explain the basic facts regarding HIV and hepatitis infection

Multiple Choice

1. How does the human immunodeficiency virus (HIV) affect the body?
   (A) It reduces blood supply to the brain.
   (B) It causes hearing impairment by damaging the inner ear.
   (C) It causes diabetes in otherwise healthy people.
   (D) It weakens the immune system so that the body cannot fight infection.

2. Which of the following is true of hepatitis B (HBV)?
   (A) HBV is caused by fecal-oral contamination.
   (B) There is no vaccine for HBV.
   (C) HBV is caused by jaundice.
   (D) HBV can be transmitted through blood or needles that are contaminated with the virus.

3. Employers must offer a free vaccine to protect HHAs from
   (A) AIDS
   (B) Hepatitis B
   (C) Hepatitis C
   (D) All bloodborne diseases

10. Identify high-risk behaviors that allow the spread of HIV

True or False

1. ____ A person is at risk for HIV or AIDS if he hugs an HIV-positive person.
2. ____ One way to protect against the spread of HIV or AIDS is to never share needles.
3. ____ Abstinence means having sex with only one person.
4. ____ A person is at risk for HIV if he has unprotected sex with an infected person.
5. ____ There are no medications that can lower the risk of getting HIV.
6. ____ Having sexual contact with many partners puts a person at a high risk for HIV.
7. ____ PEP (post-exposure prophylaxis) is a medication that cures HIV.

11. Demonstrate knowledge of the legal aspects of HIV, including testing

Short Answer

1. Why may the right to confidentiality be especially important to people who have HIV or AIDS?

____

____

____

____

2. What are two facts regarding HIV testing?

____

____

____

____

12. Identify community resources and services available to clients with HIV or AIDS

Short Answer

1. What are three types of services that might be available for people who have HIV or AIDS?

____

____

____

____

____

2. What should an HHA do if she feels that a client with HIV/AIDS needs more help?

____

____

13. Explain tuberculosis and list infection prevention guidelines

Multiple Choice

1. Tuberculosis may be transmitted
   (A) By coughing
   (B) By dancing
   (C) By wearing gloves
   (D) Through an N95 respirator
2. Tuberculosis is
   (A) A bloodborne disease
   (B) An airborne disease
   (C) A noninfectious disease
   (D) An untreatable disease
3. Someone with latent TB infection
   (A) Shows symptoms
   (B) Becomes unresponsive almost immediately
   (C) Cannot infect others
   (D) Can infect others

4. A person with TB disease
   (A) Can infect others
   (B) Does not show symptoms
   (C) Cannot be cured
   (D) Cannot infect others

5. TB disease is more likely to develop in people
   (A) Who live in rural areas
   (B) With a family history of TB
   (C) Who have weakened immune systems
   (D) Who work alone

6. The word *resistant* in multidrug-resistant TB (MDR-TB) means that
   (A) Medications can no longer kill the specific bacteria
   (B) The infected person does not want to treat his disease
   (C) Doctors do not know what causes the disease
   (D) The infected person will die from the disease

14. Explain the importance of reporting a possible exposure to an airborne or bloodborne disease

Short Answer

How does an HHA report possible exposure to an airborne or bloodborne disease?

____

____

____

____

15. Discuss MRSA, VRE, and C. *difficile*

True or False

1. ____ Methicillin-resistant *Staphylococcus aureus* (MRSA) is almost always spread by direct physical contact.

2. ____ Once a person has a vancomycin-resistant *Enterococcus* (VRE) infection, it is relatively easy to treat.

3. ____ MRSA can be spread through indirect contact by touching objects contaminated by a person with MRSA.

4. ____ Handwashing will not help control the spread of MRSA.

5. ____ VRE causes life-threatening infections in people with compromised immune systems.

6. ____ Frequent handwashing can help prevent the spread of VRE.

7. ____ Proper handwashing and handling of contaminated wastes can help prevent *Clostridioides difficile* (*C. difficile*).

8. ____ Increasing the use of antibiotics helps lower the risk of developing *C. difficile* diarrhea.

9. ____ Using hand sanitizers and washing hands with soap and water are considered equally effective when dealing with *C. difficile*.

16. List employer and employee responsibilities for infection prevention

Short Answer

Read the following and mark ER *for employer or* EE *for employee to show who is responsible for infection prevention.*

1. ____ Immediately report any exposure to infection, blood, or other body fluids

2. ____ Provide PPE for use and training on how to properly use it

3. ____ Follow all agency policies and procedures

4. ____ Take advantage of the hepatitis B vaccination

5. ____ Provide continuing in-service education on infection prevention

6. ____ Establish infection prevention procedures and an exposure control plan

7. ____ Follow client care plans and assignments

8. ____ Participate in annual education programs covering infection prevention

9. ____ Use PPE as indicated or as appropriate

10. ____ Provide free hepatitis B vaccinations

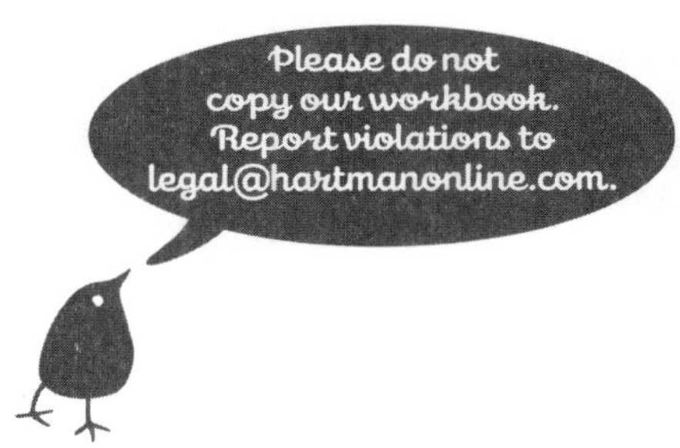

Name: ______________________________

6
Safety and Body Mechanics

1. Explain the principles of body mechanics

Labeling

Complete the illustration by labeling each part with the words listed below.

Alignment
Base of support
Center of gravity
Fulcrum
Lever

1. ______________________

2. ______________________

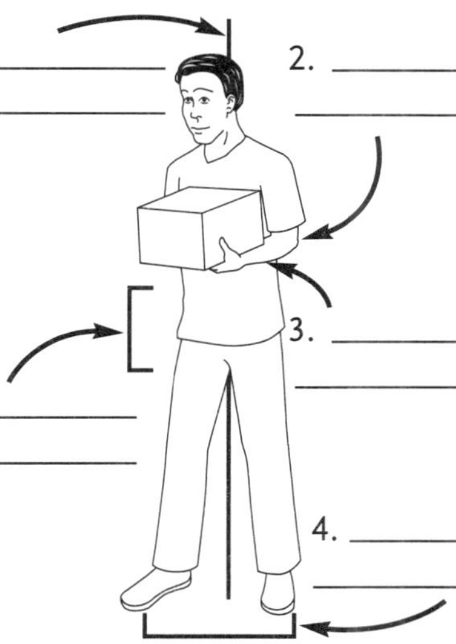

3. ______________________

5. ______________________

4. ______________________

2. Apply principles of body mechanics to daily activities

Short Answer

1. Looking at the illustrations in the next column, which drawing shows the correct way to lift objects? Why is it correct?

____

____

____

____

____

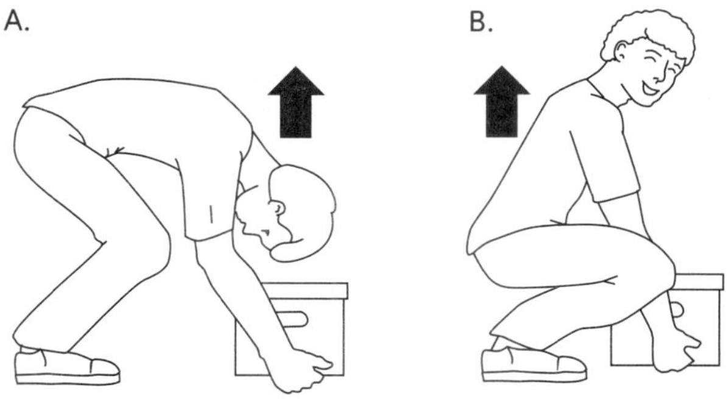

True or False

2. ____ Back injury is a serious problem that HHAs face.
3. ____ Using proper body mechanics can help save energy and prevent injury.
4. ____ When lifting an object, it is safer to hold it far away from the body.
5. ____ Feet should be pointed toward the object that a person is lifting.
6. ____ Keeping the feet close together gives the body the best base of support and keeps a person more stable.
7. ____ Lifting objects is safer than pushing objects.
8. ____ Knees should be bent when helping a client stand up.
9. ____ Twisting at the waist when lifting an object is safer than turning the entire body.

Name: ______________________________

3. List ways to adapt the home to principles of proper body mechanics

Multiple Choice

1. How should an HHA reach an object on a high shelf?
   (A) Stand on her tiptoes
   (B) Use a step stool
   (C) Climb on the closest counter
   (D) Use an umbrella

2. When sitting for long periods of time, legs should not be crossed because
   (A) It disrupts the alignment of the body
   (B) It can wrinkle a person's clothing
   (C) It is unprofessional
   (D) HHAs must stand while working

3. To be more comfortable doing tasks that require standing for long periods of time, an HHA can
   (A) Sit down every 5 minutes
   (B) Hop on one foot
   (C) Jump up and down
   (D) Place one foot on a footrest

4. Frequently used tools and supplies should be placed
   (A) On shelves or counters where they are easy to reach
   (B) On the floor to reduce the need for straining to reach
   (C) In boxes where they will be out of the way
   (D) In the attic

5. To clean a bathtub, an HHA should
   (A) Bend over
   (B) Stand upright
   (C) Kneel
   (D) Sit inside the tub

4. Identify five common types of accidents in the home

Labeling

1. In the following illustrations, circle everything that you can find that is unsafe.

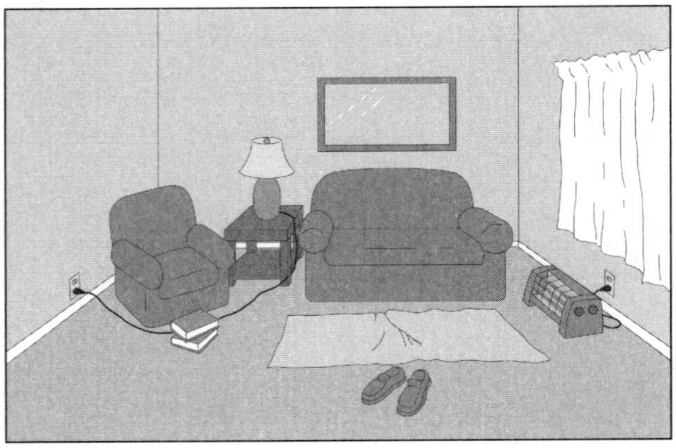

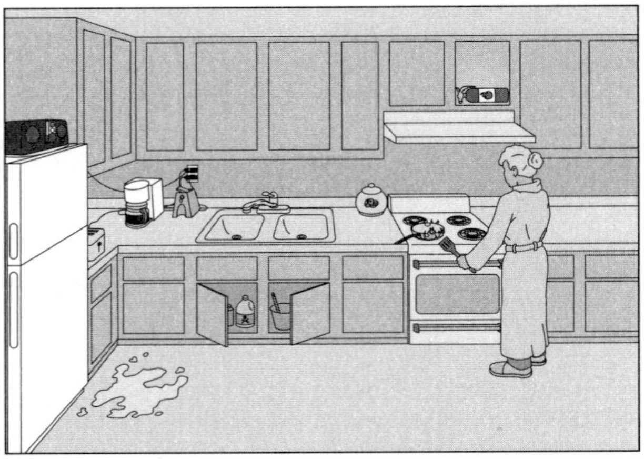

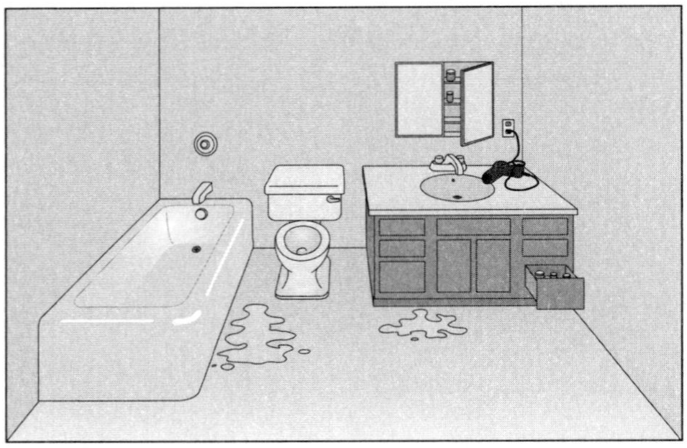

True or False

2. ____ Adjustable beds should be raised to their highest position each time the HHA has finished with care.

3. ____ Older people are often more seriously injured by falls because their bones are more fragile.

4. ____ Older adults or people with loss of sensation due to paralysis or diabetes are at the greatest risk of burns.

5. ____ Clients should be sitting down before hot drinks are served to help prevent scalds.

6. ____ Infants should sleep on their backs to prevent sudden infant death syndrome (SIDS).

7. ____ To avoid choking, clients should eat in a slightly reclined position.

8. ____ To promote safety in the kitchen, pot handles should be turned toward the back of the stove.

9. ____ A client who is ill and weak should not be left alone in a tub.

10. ____ Keeping the floor free from clutter and electrical cords helps prevent falls.

5. List home fire safety guidelines and describe what to do in case of fire

Short Answer

1. List four things that could be fire hazards.

____

____

____

____

____

____

____

____

2. What is important to remember about clothing while working near the stove?

____

____

____

____

____

3. How often should the smoke alarm be checked?

____

4. RACE is an acronym that stands for

R: ______________________________

A: ______________________________

C: ______________________________

E: ______________________________

5. PASS is an acronym that stands for

P: ______________________________

A: ______________________________

S: ______________________________

S: ______________________________

6. Explain the fire safety technique "stop, drop, and roll."

____

____

____

____

____

____

____

____

6. Identify ways to reduce the risk of automobile accidents

Multiple Choice

1. When driving to a new client's house, an HHA should
   (A) Study the map while driving there
   (B) Plan the route before leaving
   (C) Call the client to discuss the day's assignments beforehand
   (D) Text a friend for directions

2. While driving, it is best to
   (A) Keep eyes on the road and hands on the steering wheel
   (B) Call friends to pass the time more quickly
   (C) Drive quickly so that there will be more time at the client's home
   (D) Send text messages to confirm the day's schedule
3. When backing up in a car, the HHA should
   (A) Only use the rearview camera
   (B) Back up quickly
   (C) Check the rearview camera and turn her head to look behind her
   (D) Use her instincts to tell her if someone is behind her
4. Driving at a safe speed means
   (A) Exceeding the speed limit
   (B) Making adjustments for road or weather conditions
   (C) Driving faster if it is snowing
   (D) Going 10 miles per hour under the speed limit
5. Seat belts should always be worn because
   (A) They prevent accidents
   (B) They help protect a person if an accident occurs
   (C) They make the person look more professional
   (D) They make it safer to drive much faster

7. Identify guidelines for using a car on the job

True or False

1. ____ It is not necessary for an HHA to keep track of the miles he drives for work.
2. ____ An HHA's car should be serviced regularly.
3. ____ Proof of registration should be kept in the car at all times.
4. ____ Proof of insurance should be kept at home where it will be safe.
5. ____ Valuables should be put out of sight if they must be left in the car.
6. ____ All doors should be locked while driving and after exiting the car.

8. Identify guidelines for working in high-crime areas

Multiple Choice

1. An HHA is going to visit a client who lives in a high-crime area. She has been to this client's apartment before, but today as she drives up, she notices three men she does not know who are standing on the sidewalk in front of the client's apartment. They are watching her as she slows down in front of the client's apartment. What should the HHA do?
   (A) Ignore them and park the car
   (B) Keep driving past and use her phone to call her supervisor
   (C) Stop and ask them what they are doing in front of the client's apartment
   (D) Ask them if they know if her client is at home
2. An HHA is getting ready to leave a client's home as it begins to get dark. Her client lives in a large house on a street that is not well lit. She has parked next to the nearest street light, which is two houses down. What should she do on the way to her car?
   (A) Run to the car
   (B) Keep her keys inside her purse
   (C) Hold her purse or bag away from her body
   (D) Walk confidently and look as if she knows where she is going

7

Emergency Care and Disaster Preparation

1. Demonstrate how to recognize and respond to medical emergencies

Crossword

Across

4. Being mentally alert and having awareness of surroundings, sensations, and thoughts
6. In addition to completing an incident report, action the HHA should take after the emergency is over

Down

1. Type of wound that is considered a medical emergency
2. After assessing the situation, what the person who responds to a medical emergency must assess
3. In addition to checking for danger, noticing this is part of assessing the situation during a medical emergency
5. The opposite of opinions; they need to be reported when documenting an emergency

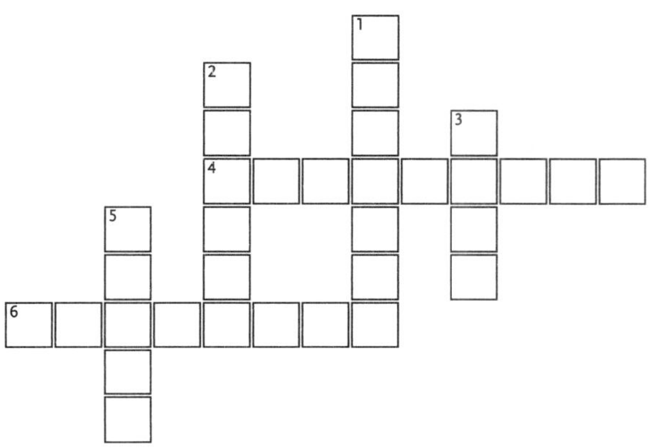

2. Demonstrate knowledge of first aid procedures

Multiple Choice

1. How can someone usually tell if a person is choking?
   (A) The choking victim will tell the person.
   (B) The choking victim will ask for food.
   (C) The choking victim will put his hands to his throat.
   (D) The choking victim will vomit.
2. How does a rescuer obtain consent to give a choking victim abdominal thrusts?
   (A) The rescuer asks the victim's spouse to sign a consent form.
   (B) The rescuer calls a family member to ask, "May I treat this person?"
   (C) The rescuer asks an attorney first.
   (D) The rescuer asks the victim, "Are you choking? I know what to do. Can I help you?"
3. Signs of shock include
   (A) Pale or bluish skin
   (B) Lack of thirst
   (C) Happiness
   (D) Relaxation
4. If an HHA suspects that a client is having a heart attack, she should
   (A) Give the client something cold to drink
   (B) Loosen the clothing around the client's neck
   (C) Encourage the client to walk around
   (D) Leave the client alone to rest

Name: ______________________________

5. To control bleeding, an HHA should
   (A) Use her bare hands to stop it
   (B) Lower the wound below the level of the heart
   (C) Hold a clean towel or cloth against the wound and press down hard
   (D) Give the client an aspirin

6. To treat a minor burn, the HHA should
   (A) Use antibacterial ointment
   (B) Use grease, such as butter
   (C) Use ice water
   (D) Use cool, clean water

7. Which of the following is true of assisting a client who is having a seizure?
   (A) The HHA should give the client a cup of water.
   (B) The HHA should hold the client down if the client is shaking.
   (C) The HHA should move furniture away to prevent injury to the client.
   (D) The HHA should open the client's mouth to move the tongue to the side.

8. If a client faints, the HHA should
   (A) Lower the client to the floor
   (B) Position the client on his side
   (C) Perform CPR
   (D) Help the client stand up immediately

9. If a client has a nosebleed, what should be the first step that the HHA takes?
   (A) Report and document the incident.
   (B) Apply pressure consistently until the bleeding stops.
   (C) Apply a cool cloth on the back of the neck, the forehead, or the upper lip.
   (D) Elevate the head of the bed or tell the client to remain in a sitting position.

10. If a client falls, the HHA should
    (A) Wait until the end of the day to assess the client before reporting the fall
    (B) Ask the client to get up and try to walk if possible
    (C) Contact her supervisor to report the fall
    (D) Begin doing range of motion exercises while the client is on the floor

3. Identify emergency evacuation procedures

Short Answer

List five ways to plan for an emergency evacuation.

____

____

____

____

____

____

____

____

____

____

4. Demonstrate knowledge of disaster procedures

Multiple Choice

1. A disaster kit should be assembled before disaster strikes. Disaster supplies include
   (A) A change of clothing
   (B) A television set
   (C) Cosmetics and a hair dryer
   (D) Three pairs of shoes

2. In a disaster, an HHA can stay informed by
   (A) Driving to a store to buy a newspaper
   (B) Going outside to talk to the client's neighbors
   (C) Listening to a radio
   (D) Calling FEMA (the Federal Emergency Management Agency)

3. If a disaster is forecast, an HHA can be prepared by
   (A) Doing her laundry
   (B) Cleaning her house
   (C) Knowing how to start a fire
   (D) Wearing appropriate clothing and shoes

4. In the event of a tornado, it is best to
   (A) Seek shelter inside a steel-framed or concrete building
   (B) Stand flat against the wall next to the windows
   (C) Seek shelter in a mobile home
   (D) Seek shelter outside in a tree or bush

5. In case of lightning, it is best to
   (A) Find water and stay in the water
   (B) Stand by the largest tree in the area
   (C) Stand underneath a tall metal object
   (D) Seek shelter in a building

6. In case of floods, it is best to
   (A) Fill the bathtub with fresh water
   (B) Drink flood water to stay hydrated
   (C) Put electrical equipment in flood water to avoid fires
   (D) Turn off the gas by yourself

7. In case of earthquakes, it is best to
   (A) Stand on a tall piece of furniture to get as high as possible
   (B) Go outside to find the closest tall building
   (C) Stop under an overpass if in a car until the shaking stops
   (D) Get under a sturdy piece of furniture

8. In an active shooter or assailant situation, it is best to
   (A) Immediately attack the shooter/assailant
   (B) Keep your phone ringer on in case police or family members need to contact you
   (C) Evacuate if there is an escape path
   (D) Try to persuade the shooter/assailant to leave

Name: ______________________________

8

Physical, Psychological, and Social Health

1. Identify basic human needs

Short Answer

1. List five basic physiological needs that all humans have.

____

____

____

____

____

____

2. List six psychosocial needs that humans have.

____

____

____

____

____

____

3. Complete your own hierarchy of needs below. Some of the examples have already been completed for you.

Maslow's Hierarchy of Needs

Need

(A) Need for self-actualization
(B) Need for self-esteem
(C) Need for love
(D) Safety and security needs
(E) Physiological needs

Example of Need

(A) I need the chance to learn new things.
(B) I need to know that I am doing a good job.
(C) ______________________________
____
____
(D) ______________________________
____
____
(E) ______________________________
____
____

True or False

4. ____ Elderly people do not have sexual needs.

5. ____ The ability to engage in sexual activity continues unless disease or injury prevents it.

6. ____ Clients have the legal right to choose how to express their sexuality.

7. ____ All elderly people usually have the same sexual behavior and desires.

8. ____ The HHA should always knock and wait for a response before entering a client's bedroom.

9. ____ If an HHA encounters a sexual situation between consenting adults, he should ask them to stop and wait until he is no longer in the home.

10. ____ If a client identifies as nonbinary and prefers the pronouns they/them, the care team should use those pronouns.

Name: ____________________________

Matching

Use each letter only once.

11. _____ Asexual
12. _____ Bisexual, bi
13. _____ Cisgender, cis
14. _____ Coming out
15. _____ Gay
16. _____ Gender identity
17. _____ Lesbian
18. _____ LGBTQ
19. _____ Nonbinary, genderqueer
20. _____ Pansexual
21. _____ Queer
22. _____ Straight
23. _____ Sexual orientation
24. _____ Transgender, trans
25. _____ Transition

(A) Acronym for lesbian, gay, bisexual, transgender, and queer

(B) A person whose physical, emotional, and/or romantic attraction is for people of a sex different from their own

(C) A person's physical, emotional, and/or romantic attraction to another person

(D) A person whose physical, emotional, and/or romantic attraction may be for people of the same gender or a different gender

(E) A person whose gender identity matches their sex assigned at birth

(F) A person whose gender identity differs from their birth sex (sex assigned at birth)

(G) A deeply felt sense of one's gender

(H) A term used to describe sexual orientation that is not exclusively straight; may not be accepted by everyone within the LGBTQ community

(I) A person whose physical, emotional, and/or romantic attraction is for people of the same sex

(J) A person who does not experience sexual attraction

(K) A person whose gender identity does not fit into the category of man or woman; the person's gender may be in between those two categories or may be entirely different from them

(L) The process of changing genders, which can include legal procedures, medical measures, and measures such as telling others and using new pronouns

(M) A woman whose physical, emotional, and/or romantic attraction is for other women

(N) A continual process of revealing one's sexual orientation or gender identity to others

(O) A person whose physical, emotional, and/or romantic attraction is for another person of any sex or gender identity

2. Define holistic care

Short Answer

In your own words, briefly describe holistic care and person-centered care.

____

____

____

____

____

____

____

____

____

____

____

____

____

3. Identify ways to help clients meet their spiritual needs

Short Answer

Place a check mark (✓) next to examples of appropriate ways to help clients with their spiritual needs.

1. ____ A client tells his HHA that he cannot drink milk with his hamburger due to his religious beliefs. He asks for some water instead. The HHA takes the milk away and brings him some water.
2. ____ A client tells her HHA that she is a Baptist and wants to know when the next Baptist service will be. The HHA asks, "Why don't you just attend a Catholic service instead? I'm Catholic, and my church is close by."
3. ____ A client asks his HHA to read a passage from his Bible. The HHA opens the Bible and begins to read.
4. ____ A client wants to see a rabbi. His HHA calls the rabbi he wants to see.
5. ____ An HHA sees a Buddha statue in a client's bedroom. The HHA chuckles and tells the client, "This little guy is so cute."
6. ____ A spiritual leader is visiting with a client. The HHA leaves the room and quietly shuts the door.
7. ____ A client tells his HHA that he is Muslim. The HHA begins to explain Christianity to him and asks him to attend a Christian service just to see what it is like.
8. ____ A client tells her HHA that she does not believe in God. The HHA does believe in God but does not argue with the client. The HHA listens quietly as the client explains her reasoning.

4. Discuss family roles and their significance in health care

Multiple Choice

Read each description below. Choose the term that best defines the type of family that is being described.

1. Mr. Dane's wife died giving birth to their twin girls. Mr. Dane never remarried and raised the girls himself.
   (A) Single-parent family
   (B) Nuclear family
   (C) Blended family
   (D) Extended family
2. Ms. Cone has lived with her best friend, Ms. Lawrence, since they graduated from college together. They both dated many men throughout their lives but were never married. Ms. Cone has a teenaged daughter who was raised in their household.
   (A) Single-parent family
   (B) Nuclear family
   (C) Blended family
   (D) Extended family
3. Mrs. Rose had three children with her first husband. She divorced him when their youngest child was 2 years old. Two years later she remarried, and she and her second husband raised her three children as well as one child from his first marriage.
   (A) Single-parent family
   (B) Nuclear family
   (C) Blended family
   (D) Extended family
4. Mrs. Parker was married to her husband for 30 years. They lived together with their two children.
   (A) Single-parent family
   (B) Nuclear family
   (C) Blended family
   (D) Extended family
5. Mr. Nicholson has been with his husband for 10 years. Their 5-year-old son lives with them.
   (A) Single-parent family
   (B) Nuclear family
   (C) Blended family
   (D) Extended family

Name: ______________________________

5. Describe personal adjustments of the individual and family to illness and disability

Short Answer

List three adjustments that family members may need to make due to a client's illness or disability.

____

____

____

____

____

____

____

____

____

____

____

____

____

____

____

____

____

6. Identify community resources for individual and family health

Short Answer

If an HHA believes that a client needs help finding community resources, what should he do?

____

____

____

____

7. List ways to respond to emotional needs of clients and their families

Multiple Choice

1. An HHA arrives at her client's house to find the client's wife, Mrs. McNabb, upset and close to tears. She tells the HHA that her husband simply will not eat his breakfast. When the HHA asks what she served him for breakfast, Mrs. McNabb begins to cry. What would be the best response by the HHA?
   (A) The HHA should ask her not to cry.
   (B) The HHA should ask her why she is crying over something so unimportant.
   (C) The HHA should reassure her that the HHA is there to help.
   (D) The HHA should tell Mrs. McNabb that her reaction is probably increasing her stress level.

2. The HHA encourages Mrs. McNabb to talk about what is bothering her. Mrs. McNabb confesses that she is feeling very overwhelmed. What would be the best response by the HHA?
   (A) "I know just how you feel. My kids are a handful, too."
   (B) "It sounds like you are under a lot of stress. Can I help in some way?"
   (C) "Well, I work two jobs myself, and it's no big deal."
   (D) "I think attending church services more often would help you."

3. Mrs. McNabb asks if the HHA can stay longer to help her out with the cooking and cleaning. What would be the best response by the HHA?
   (A) "I'll talk to my supervisor and see what she says. Maybe we can work something out."
   (B) "You can call a cleaning service for help."
   (C) "That's not in my job description."
   (D) "If you will pay me extra money, I can consider it."

9

Body Systems and Related Conditions

1. Describe the integumentary system and related conditions

Fill in the Blank

1. The largest organ and system in the body is the ______________________.
2. Skin prevents ______________________ to internal organs.
3. Skin also prevents the loss of too much ____________, which is essential to life.
4. The skin is also a ____________ organ that feels heat, cold, pain, touch, and pressure.
5. Blood vessels ______________________, or widen, when the outside temperature is too high.
6. Blood vessels ______________________, or narrow, when the outside temperature is too cold.

Labeling

For each position shown, list the areas at risk for skin breakdown.

Lateral Position

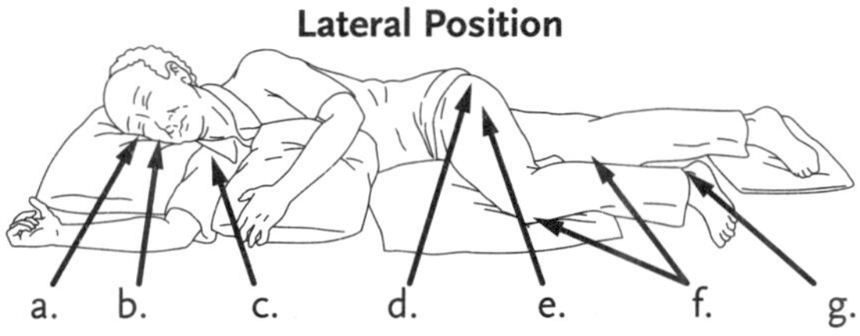

7. Lateral Position

   a. ______________________

   b. ______________________

   c. ______________________

   d. ______________________

   e. ______________________

   f. ______________________

   g. ______________________

Prone Position

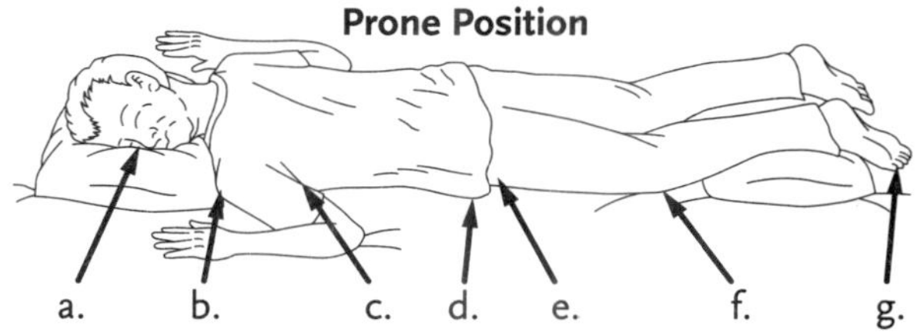

8. Prone Position

   a. ______________________

   b. ______________________

   c. ______________________

   d. ______________________

   e. ______________________

   f. ______________________

   g. ______________________

Supine Position

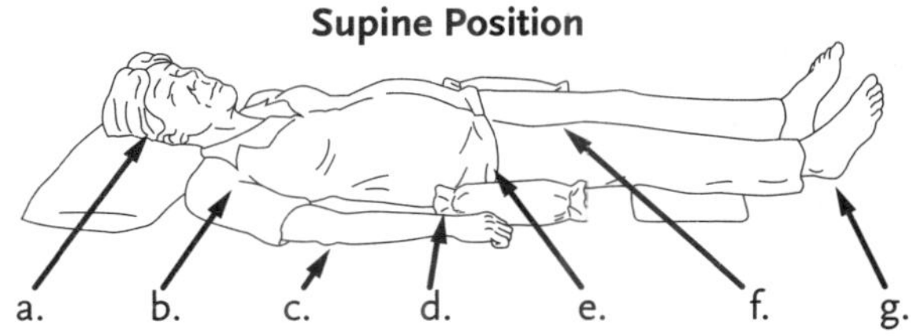

9. Supine Position

   a. ______________________

   b. ______________________

   c. ______________________

   d. ______________________

   e. ______________________

   f. ______________________

   g. ______________________

Name: ____________________

True or False

10. ____ With a stage 1 pressure injury, skin is intact but may be red or a different color than the surrounding area.
11. ____ Pressure injuries usually occur in areas of the body where bone lies close to the skin.
12. ____ An older name for pressure injuries is decubitus ulcers.
13. ____ Common sites for pressure injuries are the chest, nose, and hands.
14. ____ A contusion is a type of open wound.
15. ____ An open wound has skin that is not intact.
16. ____ Stasis dermatitis is usually caused when blood pools in the legs due to poor circulation.

Matching

Use each letter only once.

17. ____ Cellulitis
18. ____ Dermatitis
19. ____ Scabies
20. ____ Shingles
21. ____ Wound

(A) A bacterial infection affecting the skin and soft tissue

(B) Contagious skin infection caused by a mite that burrows into the skin, where it lays eggs, causing intense itching and a skin rash

(C) A type of injury to the skin; classified as either closed or open

(D) Skin rash caused by the varicella-zoster virus (VZV), which is the same virus that causes chickenpox

(E) A general term that refers to an inflammation of the skin

2. Describe the musculoskeletal system and related conditions

True or False

1. ____ The body is shaped by muscles, bones, ligaments, tendons, and cartilage.
2. ____ The human body has 215 bones.
3. ____ Bones protect the body's organs.
4. ____ Two bones meet at a joint.
5. ____ Muscles provide movement of body parts.
6. ____ Range of motion exercises help prevent problems related to immobility.

Multiple Choice

7. Arthritis is a general term referring to ______ of the joints.
   (A) Immobility
   (B) Inflammation
   (C) Redness
   (D) Stiffness

8. Pain and stiffness of osteoarthritis may increase with
   (A) Hot weather
   (B) Cold weather
   (C) An active lifestyle
   (D) Intake of fluids

9. Arthritis is generally treated with
   (A) Botox
   (B) Plastic surgery
   (C) Deep breathing exercises
   (D) Anti-inflammatory medications

10. Rheumatoid arthritis (RA) affects the ____________ joints first.
    (A) Smaller
    (B) Larger
    (C) Elbow
    (D) There is no typical progression.

Complete the Sentence

11. Muscular dystrophy (MD) is an *autoimmune* | *inherited* disease that causes gradual wasting away of the muscles.
12. Most forms of MD become apparent in *middle adulthood* | *infancy or childhood.*

13. People with amyotrophic lateral sclerosis (ALS) usually live *2 to 5* | *more than 10* years after diagnosis.

14. Osteoporosis causes bones to become *dense and strong* | *porous and brittle.*

15. Phantom limb pain occurs when a person feels pain in a limb or extremity that *is affected by an illness* | *has been amputated.*

3. Describe the nervous system and related conditions

Multiple Choice

1. The nervous system
   (A) Gives the body shape and structure
   (B) Controls and coordinates body function
   (C) Is the largest organ in the body
   (D) Pumps blood through the blood vessels to the cells

2. The basic unit of the nervous system is the
   (A) Neuron
   (B) Message
   (C) Brain
   (D) Spinal cord

3. The two main parts of the nervous system are
   (A) The cardiovascular system and integumentary system
   (B) Neurons and receptors
   (C) The body and the brain
   (D) The central nervous system and peripheral nervous system

4. The central nervous system (CNS) is made up of
   (A) The brain and spinal cord
   (B) Muscles and bones
   (C) Neurons and receptors
   (D) The heart and lungs

5. The peripheral nervous system (PNS) deals with the outer part of the body and conducts messages to the brain through the
   (A) Limbs
   (B) Cerebrum
   (C) Nerves
   (D) Right hemisphere

True or False

Mark each of the following statements regarding CVA (stroke) with either a T *for true or an* F *for false.*

6. ____ Clients with paralysis or loss of movement will not need physical therapy.

7. ____ Range of motion exercises strengthen muscles and keep joints mobile.

8. ____ When helping with transfers or ambulation, the HHA should stand on the client's stronger side.

9. ____ The HHA should always use a transfer belt for safety when helping a client who has had a stroke with transfers.

10. ____ Gestures and facial expressions are important in communicating with a client who has had a stroke.

11. ____ Food should always be placed in the unaffected, or stronger, side of the mouth.

12. ____ When assisting with dressing a client who has had a stroke, the HHA should dress the stronger side first.

Short Answer

Read each of the following scenarios about Kate, an HHA, caring for Mr. Manhas who is recovering from a stroke. Then answer the questions.

13. Kate, an HHA, is getting ready to prepare lunch for Mr. Manhas. Mr. Manhas has difficulty communicating and also suffers from confusion. "Let's see," Kate says. "For lunch we can have soup, sandwiches, some leftover casserole, or I can make a salad. Now, what would you like to eat?" What is wrong with the way Kate is communicating with Mr. Manhas?

____

____

____

____

____

____

____

Name: ______________________________

14. Mr. Manhas's wife comes home after running some errands and asks how her husband is doing. As she and Kate walk into the kitchen where Mr. Manhas is sitting, Kate says, "Mr. Manhas is having trouble today with his eating. Just look at him. He's spilled food all over himself." What is wrong with what Kate has just said?

____

____

____

____

____

____

____

____

15. Kate notices that Mr. Manhas seems to be having trouble saying words clearly. He is beginning to get frustrated because he cannot tell Kate what he wants. Kate decides to ask only yes or no questions, so she tells Mr. Manhas, "If you find it too difficult to speak right now, why don't you try nodding your head for 'yes' and shaking your head for 'no'?" What is Kate doing right?

____

____

____

____

____

____

____

True or False

Mark each of the following statements regarding Parkinson disease with either a T *for true or an* F *for false.*

16. ____ Parkinson disease puts a person at a high risk for falls.

17. ____ Parkinson disease causes a shuffling gait and a masklike facial expression.

18. ____ Pill-rolling is something that people with Parkinson disease must do before taking their medication.

19. ____ Clients with Parkinson disease should be discouraged from performing their own care to save their energy.

Fill in the Blank

Fill in the blanks for each of the following statements regarding multiple sclerosis (MS).

20. For a person who has MS, nerves cannot send ______________________ to and from the brain in a normal way.

21. Symptoms of MS include ______________ vision, fatigue, tremors, poor balance, and difficulty walking.

22. The HHA should offer ______________________ periods as necessary for clients with MS.

23. The HHA should give clients plenty of time to ______________________ because people with MS often have trouble forming their thoughts.

24. ______________________ can worsen the effects of MS, so the HHA should remain calm and listen to clients when they want to talk.

Complete the Sentence

In each of the following sentences about head and spinal cord injuries, underline the correct choice between the words or phrases in italics.

25. The effects of a spinal cord injury depend on the force of impact and the *location* | *time* of the injury.

26. The lower the injury on the spinal cord, the *less* | *greater* the loss of function will be.

27. *Quadriplegia* | *Paraplegia* is the loss of function of the lower body and legs.

28. Clients with head or spinal cord injuries will need *emotional support* | *all decisions made for them* as well as physical help.

29. People with spinal cord injuries may not *be able to smell or taste | feel burns* because of loss of sensation.

30. The HHA should help clients change positions at least every *2 hours | half hour* to prevent pressure injuries.

Multiple Choice

Circle the letter of the answer that best completes the statement regarding hearing impairment.

31. To best communicate with a client who has a hearing impairment, the HHA should
    (A) Use short sentences and simple words
    (B) Shout words slowly
    (C) Approach the client from behind
    (D) Raise the pitch of her voice

32. If a client is difficult to understand, the HHA should
    (A) Pretend to understand the client so as not to hurt his feelings
    (B) Mouth the words in an exaggerated way so that the client will mimic that behavior next time
    (C) Ask the client to repeat what he said, and then tell the client what the HHA thinks she heard
    (D) Ask the client to shout

Matching

For each of the following terms regarding vision impairment, write the letter of the correct definition from the list below. Use each letter only once.

33. _____ Age-related macular degeneration (AMD)

34. _____ Cataract

35. _____ Diabetic retinopathy

36. _____ Glaucoma

37. _____ Hyperopia (farsightedness)

38. _____ Myopia (nearsightedness)

(A) _____ Condition that causes increased pressure in the eye and may cause blindness

(B) _____ The ability to see objects in the distance better than objects nearby

(C) _____ Condition that causes cloudiness of the lens of the eye, which can cause loss of vision

(D) _____ The ability to see objects that are nearby better than objects in the distance

(E) _____ Condition that causes a person to see spots or have blurred vision and makes it hard to see well at night

(F) _____ Condition that occurs when part of the retina gradually deteriorates, affecting the ability to recognize faces, drive, read, and write

4. Describe the circulatory system and related conditions

Multiple Choice

1. The two lower chambers of the heart are called the
    (A) Atria
    (B) Cells
    (C) Ventricles
    (D) Pericardia

2. What functions as the pump of the circulatory system?
    (A) Heart
    (B) Lungs
    (C) Lymph
    (D) Blood

3. What occurs during the resting phase, or diastole?
    (A) Ventricles pump blood through the blood vessels.
    (B) The heart begins beating rapidly until the next contraction.
    (C) Circulation stops.
    (D) The chambers fill with blood.

4. Which of the following is one of the functions that the circulatory system performs?
    (A) Senses and interprets information from the environment
    (B) Supplies nutrients, oxygen, and hormones to cells
    (C) Adds waste products to the cells
    (D) Processes carbohydrates and proteins to meet the body's energy needs

Name: ______________________________

Matching

Use each letter only once.

5. ____ Angina
6. ____ Atherosclerosis
7. ____ Deep vein thrombosis
8. ____ Diuretic
9. ____ Heart failure
10. ____ Hypertension
11. ____ Myocardial infarction
12. ____ Nitroglycerin

(A) Condition in which the heart fails to pump effectively, causing blood to back up into the lungs or the legs, feet, or abdomen

(B) Medical term for high blood pressure

(C) Chest pain, pressure, or discomfort

(D) Medication that relaxes the walls of the coronary arteries, allowing them to open and get more blood to the heart

(E) Condition in which blood flow to the heart muscle is blocked and the muscle cells die

(F) Medications that reduce fluid in the body

(G) Hardening and narrowing of the blood vessels

(H) Occurs when a blood clot forms in the limbs or pelvis; can cause pulmonary embolism

5. Describe the respiratory system and related conditions

Fill in the Blank

1. Respiration is the body taking in ____________________ and removing ____________ ____________.

2. Respiration involves breathing in, or ____________________, and breathing out, or ____________________.

3. The ______________________________ accomplish the process of respiration.

Multiple Choice

4. Clients with chronic obstructive pulmonary disease (COPD) have difficulty with
   (A) Breathing
   (B) Urination
   (C) Losing weight
   (D) Vision

5. The best position for a client with COPD is
   (A) Lying flat on his back
   (B) Sitting upright
   (C) Lying on his stomach
   (D) Lying on his side

6. Part of the HHA's role in caring for a client with COPD includes
   (A) Being calm and supportive
   (B) Adjusting oxygen levels
   (C) Making changes in the client's diet
   (D) Doing everything for the client as much as possible

7. Emphysema usually develops as a result of
   (A) Cigarette smoking
   (B) Alcohol use
   (C) Radiation therapy
   (D) Excessive weight loss

8. Chronic bronchitis and emphysema are grouped under
   (A) Chronic obstructive pulmonary disease, or COPD
   (B) Muscular dystrophy, or MD
   (C) Hypertension, or HTN
   (D) Coronary artery disease, or CAD

9. Bronchitis is usually caused by
   (A) Bacteria
   (B) Exposure to cold weather
   (C) Environmental toxins
   (D) A virus

10. Which of the following types of PPE should always be used when caring for a client with COVID-19?
   (A) Mask or respirator
   (B) Shoe covering
   (C) Gown
   (D) Hazmat suit

11. Which of the following can worsen asthma?
    (A) Warm air humidifier
    (B) Exercise
    (C) Hot water bottle
    (D) Electric heating pad

12. An upper respiratory infection (URI) is most often treated by
    (A) Rest and fluids
    (B) A ventilator
    (C) Occupational therapy
    (D) Intravenous infusions

6. Describe the urinary system and related conditions

Short Answer

1. List two vital functions of the urinary system.

____

____

____

____

____

2. What is one reason why women are more likely than men to have urinary tract infections?

____

____

____

____

____

3. In which direction should clients wipe after elimination to help avoid a urinary tract infection (UTI)?

____

____

____

Multiple Choice

4. Which of the following statements is true of urinary incontinence?
    (A) It is a normal part of getting older.
    (B) It is a risk factor for pressure injuries.
    (C) Drinking plenty of fluids makes the problem worse.
    (D) It is treated by using inhalers and doing deep breathing exercises.

5. Clients who are __________ are more likely to have urinary incontinence.
    (A) Bedbound
    (B) Active
    (C) Vegetarians
    (D) Strong

6. What can clients do to help prevent urinary tract infections?
    (A) Limit their fluid intake
    (B) Increase their fluid intake
    (C) Increase their fiber intake
    (D) Avoid cleaning the perineal area

True or False

7. ____ *Nephrolithiasis* is the medical term for chronic kidney disease.

8. ____ Kidney failure is fatal without proper treatment.

9. ____ In one form of dialysis, a solution is instilled in the abdomen and the lining of the peritoneum filters the blood.

10. ____ High levels of salt in the diet promote kidney health.

7. Describe the gastrointestinal system and related conditions

Crossword

Across

2. Position that the body should be in during sleep if the client has heartburn or gastroesophageal reflux disease

6. Disorder that occurs from decreased fluid intake, poor diet/lack of fiber, inactivity, medications, aging, certain diseases, or ignoring the urge to eliminate

Name: ______________________

8. Process of expelling wastes (made up of the waste products of food and fluids) that are not absorbed into the cells

Down

1. Abbreviation for gastroesophageal reflux disease
3. Another name for the digestive system
4. The process of preparing food physically and chemically so that it can be absorbed into the cells
5. Artificial opening through the abdomen to which waste is diverted
7. Adding this into the diet may help treat hemorrhoids

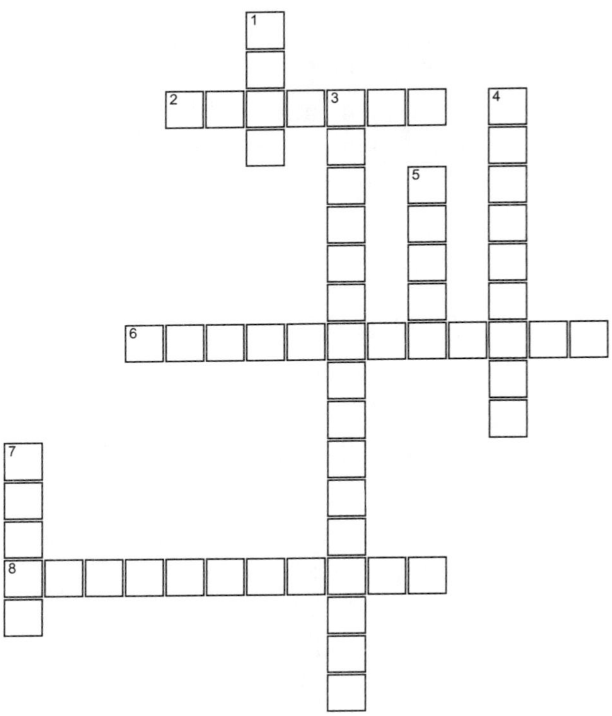

Multiple Choice

9. When a client has gastroesophageal reflux disease, it is best for the client not to lie down until at least _____ hours after eating.
   (A) 2
   (B) 6
   (C) 4
   (D) 8

10. These may be caused by excessive acid secretion:
   (A) Nausea and vomiting
   (B) Diarrhea and dehydration
   (C) Peptic ulcers
   (D) Heartburn and constipation

11. Irritable bowel syndrome (IBS) is the result of
   (A) Problems in communication between the nervous system and digestive tract
   (B) Physical damage caused to the small intestine
   (C) Colorectal cancer
   (D) Poor diet

12. Two different illnesses are forms of inflammatory bowel disease (IBD):
   (A) IBS and Crohn disease
   (B) Crohn disease and ulcerative colitis
   (C) GERD and heartburn
   (D) Fecal impaction and GERD

8. Describe the endocrine system and related conditions

Fill in the Blank

1. The endocrine system is made up of ______________________ in different areas of the body.
2. Chemical substances created by the body that control numerous body functions are called ______________________.
3. One function of the endocrine system is to regulate levels of phosphate and ______________________.

Multiple Choice

4. Diabetes is a condition in which the pancreas does not produce any, enough, or does not properly use
   (A) Insulin
   (B) Glucose
   (C) Growth hormones
   (D) Adrenaline

5. Sugars collecting in the blood cause problems with
   (A) Breathing
   (B) Circulation
   (C) Pain level
   (D) Ambulation

6. Type 1 diabetes
   (A) Continues throughout a person's life
   (B) Is most common in the elderly
   (C) Is first treated with surgery
   (D) Does not require a change of diet

7. Changes in the circulatory system from diabetes can cause
   (A) Hair loss
   (B) Heart attack and stroke
   (C) Multiple sclerosis
   (D) COPD

8. The most common form of diabetes is
   (A) Insulin reaction
   (B) Gestational diabetes
   (C) Type 1 diabetes
   (D) Type 2 diabetes

9. Poor circulation and impaired wound healing may result in
   (A) Urinary tract infections
   (B) Cancer
   (C) Leg and foot ulcers
   (D) An autoimmune disease

10. Gangrene can lead to
    (A) Loss of bowel control
    (B) Peripheral vascular disease
    (C) Heart failure
    (D) Amputation

11. What condition occurs when a person's blood glucose level is above normal but not high enough for a diagnosis of type 2 diabetes?
    (A) Gestational diabetes
    (B) Type 1 diabetes
    (C) Prediabetes
    (D) Hyperglycemia

12. Careful ________ care is especially important for people with diabetes.
    (A) Foot
    (B) Hair
    (C) Facial
    (D) Mouth

13. Diabetes can lead to the following complication:
    (A) Hypoglycemia
    (B) Mastectomy
    (C) Cancer
    (D) Arthritis

14. What type of shoe material is best for people who have diabetes because the material helps prevent a buildup of moisture?
    (A) Plastic
    (B) Cotton
    (C) Rubber
    (D) Metal

15. For a client who has diabetes, where should lotion not be applied?
    (A) Upper arms
    (B) Lower back
    (C) Back of the legs
    (D) Between the toes

16. The meal plan for a client with diabetes may involve
    (A) Counting carbohydrates
    (B) Eating more sugary items
    (C) Fasting for long periods to get blood glucose levels near normal
    (D) Eating fatty foods to gain weight

17. Which of the following is true of an HHA's responsibilities for a client who has diabetes?
    (A) The HHA may need to inject insulin at regular times.
    (B) The HHA may assist with the client's exercise program.
    (C) The HHA will create the meal plan for the client.
    (D) The HHA needs to cut the client's toenails when giving foot care.

Name: ______________________

18. What is another name for hypoglycemia?
    (A) Sugar coma
    (B) Diabetic ketoacidosis
    (C) Insulin reaction
    (D) Diabetes

19. What is a common symptom of hypothyroidism?
    (A) Rapid heartbeat
    (B) Weight gain
    (C) High blood pressure
    (D) Bulging eyes

20. What autoimmune disorder commonly causes hyperthyroidism?
    (A) Multiple sclerosis
    (B) Graves disease
    (C) Rheumatoid arthritis
    (D) Hashimoto thyroiditis

9. Describe the reproductive system and related conditions

Multiple Choice

1. The reproductive system allows humans to
   (A) Move and speak
   (B) Create human life
   (C) Think logically
   (D) Fight disease

2. The male and female sex glands are called the
   (A) Glands
   (B) Ureters
   (C) Gonads
   (D) Urethras

3. Vaginitis may be caused by bacteria, protozoa, or
   (A) Hypertrophy
   (B) Lymph
   (C) Fungus
   (D) Discharge

4. Which of the following is a type of contact that can cause a sexually-transmitted infection (STI)?
   (A) Holding hands with an infected person
   (B) Having sexual intercourse with an infected person
   (C) Hugging an infected person
   (D) Dining with an infected person

True or False

5. ____ Genital herpes can be cured with antibiotics.

6. ____ Syphilis is caused by bacteria.

7. ____ STIs can be transmitted by contact of the mouth with the genitals of an infected person.

8. ____ There is a vaccine available for human papillomavirus (HPV).

9. ____ Benign prostatic hyperplasia (BPH) is a disorder that commonly occurs in men around age 45.

10. ____ Yeast infections are often caused by an overproduction of a fungus.

10. Describe the immune and lymphatic systems and related conditions

Short Answer

1. What is the difference between nonspecific immunity and specific immunity?

____
____
____
____
____
____
____
____

2. What two systems are related to the lymphatic system?

____
____
____

3. How is lymph fluid circulated?

____
____

Name: ______________________________

____

____

Multiple Choice

4. Care for a person who has HIV or AIDS should focus on
   (A) Helping to find a cure for HIV
   (B) Preventing visits from friends and family so as not to infect them
   (C) Providing relief of symptoms and preventing infection
   (D) Letting the person know that his life choices caused this disease

5. If a client with AIDS has a poor appetite, the HHA should
   (A) Give the client an appetite stimulant
   (B) Serve familiar and favorite foods
   (C) Let the client know that if he does not eat, he might die
   (D) Discuss this with the client's family to see what they recommend doing

6. When caring for a client with AIDS, safety guidelines for food preparation are
   (A) Important because foodborne illnesses can cause death
   (B) Important because the HHA might become infected with HIV
   (C) Important because the HHA might infect family members with HIV
   (D) Not especially important

7. Clients who have AIDS and have infections of the mouth and esophagus may need to eat food that is
   (A) Spicy
   (B) Low in acid
   (C) Dry
   (D) Very hot

8. Someone who has nausea and vomiting should
   (A) Eat mostly dairy products
   (B) Eat high-fat foods
   (C) Drink liquids and eat salty foods
   (D) Reduce liquid intake

9. Fluids are important for clients who have diarrhea because
   (A) Diarrhea rapidly depletes the body of fluids
   (B) Diarrhea can be prevented by drinking a lot of fluids
   (C) Diarrhea is an infection that can be flushed out by fluids
   (D) Diarrhea can make a client's throat dry

10. The following is helpful in dealing with neuropathy (numbness, tingling, and pain in the feet):
   (A) Wrapping the feet in bandages
   (B) Wearing tight shoes
   (C) Using a bed cradle
   (D) Tucking in bed sheets over the feet tightly

11. Discuss cancer and related care

Short Answer

Mark an X beside the American Cancer Society's warning signs of cancer.

1. ____ Change in bowel or bladder function
2. ____ Difficulty breathing
3. ____ Dizziness
4. ____ Thickening or lump in a breast
5. ____ Memory loss
6. ____ Change in appearance of a wart or mole
7. ____ Joint aches
8. ____ Nagging cough
9. ____ Indigestion or difficulty swallowing
10. ____ Nausea
11. ____ Sweet, fruity breath odor
12. ____ Sores that do not heal
13. ____ Unusual bleeding or discharge
14. ____ Headache

Name: ______________________

Multiple Choice

15. The key treatment for malignant tumors of the skin, breast, bladder, colon, rectum, stomach, and muscle is
    (A) Surgery
    (B) Homeopathic pills
    (C) Radiation
    (D) Hormone therapy

16. Nausea, vomiting, diarrhea, hair loss, and decreased resistance to infection are all side effects of which treatment?
    (A) Surgery
    (B) Chemotherapy
    (C) Diet and exercise
    (D) Herbal remedies

17. This treatment method uses medications to destroy cancer cells:
    (A) Surgery
    (B) Chemotherapy
    (C) Radiation
    (D) Herbal remedies

18. This treatment method involves removing as much of the tumor as possible to prevent cancer from spreading:
    (A) Surgery
    (B) Chemotherapy
    (C) Radiation
    (D) Hormone therapy

19. This treatment method kills normal and abnormal cells in a limited area, sometimes causing skin to become sore, irritated, or burned:
    (A) Surgery
    (B) Chemotherapy
    (C) Radiation
    (D) Immunotherapy

20. To help promote proper nutrition for a client with cancer, the HHA should do the following:
    (A) Use metal utensils when serving meals
    (B) Serve favorite foods that are high in nutrition
    (C) Restrict nutritional supplements
    (D) Serve foods with little nutritional content

21. If a client is experiencing pain, the HHA should
    (A) Assist with comfort measures
    (B) Let the client know that there is little the HHA can do
    (C) Prescribe pain medication
    (D) Give the client a shot of pain medication

22. When providing skin care, which of the following should the HHA do?
    (A) Use lotion regularly on dry skin
    (B) Remove markings that are used in radiation therapy
    (C) Clean the client's face with soap
    (D) Apply lotion to areas receiving radiation therapy

23. Which of the following should an HHA do regarding oral care for a client with cancer?
    (A) Rinse the client's mouth with a type of commercial mouthwash
    (B) Use a soft-bristled toothbrush to brush the client's teeth
    (C) Use rubbing alcohol for any mouth sores the client has
    (D) Avoid giving the client oral care

24. Which of the following should the HHA do when communicating with a client who has cancer?
    (A) Insist that the client tell the HHA what he is going through
    (B) Let the client know about any new medications that might help him
    (C) If the client is worried, tell him, "Don't worry. It will all be fine."
    (D) Listen to the client if he wishes to share his feelings

25. A condition that makes it difficult for a person with cancer to fight infection is
    (A) Obesity
    (B) Neutropenia
    (C) Neuropathy
    (D) Nonspecific immunity

10

Confusion, Dementia, and Alzheimer Disease

1. Discuss confusion and delirium

Short Answer

1. What are 10 actions that an HHA can take when helping care for a client who is confused?

____

____

____

____

____

____

____

____

____

____

____

____

2. Name four possible causes of delirium.

____

____

____

____

____

____

____

____

2. Describe dementia

Multiple Choice

1. The ability to think logically and clearly is called
   (A) Cognition
   (B) Dementia
   (C) Awareness
   (D) Respiration

2. When a person has cognitive impairment, her ________ are affected.
   (A) Blood pressure readings and ambulatory abilities
   (B) Motor skills and fine motor skills
   (C) Concentration and memory
   (D) Diet choices and exercise abilities

3. HHAs can help clients by
   (A) Doing as much as possible for them
   (B) Encouraging them to make lists of things to remember
   (C) Reminding them every time they forget something
   (D) Telling them to think as hard as they can

4. The most common cause of dementia is
   (A) Lewy body dementia
   (B) Alzheimer disease
   (C) Reproductive cancers
   (D) Chronic obstructive pulmonary disease

3. Describe Alzheimer disease and identify its stages

True or False

1. ____ A person with Alzheimer disease is usually able to continue using skills that he used often during his lifetime.

Name: ______________________

2. ____ Each person with Alzheimer disease shows the same symptoms at the same times during their lives.
3. ____ An HHA should perform as many activities as possible for clients with Alzheimer disease.
4. ____ Alzheimer disease cannot be cured.
5. ____ Most people who have Alzheimer disease will eventually be dependent on others for care.

4. Identify personal attitudes helpful in caring for clients with Alzheimer disease

Short Answer

For each of the following, briefly describe why each attitude is helpful when caring for clients with Alzheimer disease.

1. Do not take things personally.

2. Be empathetic.

3. Work with the symptoms and behaviors noted.

4. Work as a team.

5. Be aware of difficulties associated with caregiving.

6. Work with family members.

7. Remember the goals of the care plan.

5. List strategies for better communication with clients with Alzheimer disease

Short Answer

Read each scenario below and state an appropriate response.

1. Mrs. Hays, a client with AD, has awakened from her nap and does not recognize her room or anyone around her.

2. Makayla, an HHA, has been trying to give Mr. Collins, a client with AD, a bath. Mr. Collins has become agitated and is asking Makayla "Who are you?" over and over again, although Makayla has already identified herself twice.

3. Mrs. Hays has been telling Makayla a story about her niece. She is showing Makayla a necklace that her niece gave her as a gift. She is having trouble remembering the word *necklace* and is getting upset.

4. Makayla is helping Mr. Collins get ready to eat dinner with his family. Makayla asks him to put his shoes on, but Mr. Collins does not understand what Makayla wants him to do.

Multiple Choice

5. When communicating with a client with Alzheimer disease, the HHA should
   (A) Quietly approach the client from behind
   (B) Stand as close as possible to the client
   (C) Communicate in a loud area to help cheer up the client
   (D) Speak slowly, using a lower voice than normal

6. If a client is frightened or anxious, which of the following should the HHA do?
   (A) Check her body language so that she does not appear tense or hurried
   (B) Turn up the television or radio to try to distract the client
   (C) Use complex, longer sentences to calm the client
   (D) Give multiple instructions at one time so that the client has something to process

7. If a client perseverates, this means they are
   (A) Repeating words, phrases, questions, or actions
   (B) Suggesting words that sound correct
   (C) Hallucinating
   (D) Gesturing instead of speaking

8. If the client does not remember how to perform basic tasks, the HHA should
   (A) Do everything for him
   (B) Break each activity into simple steps
   (C) Skip explaining each activity
   (D) Say "don't" as often as the HHA feels is necessary

6. Explain general principles that will help assist clients with personal care

Short Answer

What three principles will help HHAs give clients with dementia the best personal care?

____

____

____

____

____

____

____

7. List and describe interventions for problems with common activities of daily living (ADLs)

Short Answer

For each of the following statements, write G *if the statement is a good idea for clients with Alzheimer disease or* B *if the statement is a bad idea.*

1. ____ Use nonslip mats, tub seats, and handholds to ensure safety during bathing.
2. ____ Break tasks down into simple steps, introducing one step at a time.
3. ____ Do not attempt to groom the client; people with Alzheimer disease usually do not care about their appearance.
4. ____ Choose clothes that are simple to put on.
5. ____ If the client has urinary incontinence, do not give her fluids.
6. ____ Mark the bathroom with a sign as a reminder of where it is.
7. ____ Check the skin regularly for signs of irritation.
8. ____ Do not encourage exercise as this will make the client more agitated.
9. ____ Serve finger foods.
10. ____ Schedule meals at the same time every day.
11. ____ Serve new kinds of foods as often as possible to stimulate the client.
12. ____ Put only one kind of food on the plate at a time.
13. ____ Use dishes with contrasting colors for serving food.
14. ____ Reward positive behavior with smiles and warm touches.

8. List and describe interventions for common difficult behaviors related to Alzheimer disease

Short Answer

For each description below, identify the behavior that the client with Alzheimer disease is exhibiting, and describe one way of dealing with it.

1. Mr. Fejer gets upset at about nine o'clock every night. He repeatedly asks for snacks or drinks and refuses to go to bed.

____

____

____

____

____

____

____

____

2. Mr. Noble is playing chess with a friend who is visiting. Mr. Noble becomes angry when he loses the game. He shoves his friend and when the HHA approaches them, he tells her he is going to hit her.

____

3. Ms. Desmond used to enjoy talking to people and reading, but lately she does not seem to enjoy anything. She sleeps most of the day and never talks to anyone unless she is asked to.

____

4. Ms. Storey is walking around asking her HHA what time it is. Even though she has been told several times, she still seems unsatisfied and keeps asking the question.

____

5. Mrs. Calderon tells her HHA that her husband just called her. She says he is coming to pick her up and they are going to dinner at the restaurant where they went on their first date. The HHA knows that her husband has been dead for several years, and their favorite restaurant has long since closed down.

____

9. Describe creative therapies for clients with Alzheimer disease

Short Answer

For each situation described below, identify the therapy that the HHA is using.

1. Ms. Lee's husband died 10 years ago and she misses him very much. Imani, an HHA who works with her, always asks about her life with her husband and what it was like. Ms. Lee seems to enjoy telling Imani stories about what they did when they were young and how happy she was when they were together.

____

2. Mr. Elking tells Imani that he has a date with Rose, the pretty girl who lives across the street. He is going to take her dancing and out to a movie. Imani knows that Rose lived in his neighborhood when he was a teenager and that he has not seen her for decades. Mr. Elking rarely gets out of bed. Instead of correcting him, Imani asks him what kind of movie they are going to see and what he thinks he should wear.

Name: ____________________

____

____

3. Mr. Tennant sometimes gets depressed, especially in the evenings. Imani knows that he loves classical music, so she starts playing it for him in the evenings a little before he usually starts feeling sad. He sorts through albums and places them in stacks.

____

____

10. Discuss how Alzheimer disease may affect the family

Short Answer

1. Why might families of people who have AD have a difficult time?

____

____

____

____

____

____

____

____

____

2. What two major resources affect the ability of clients' families to cope with AD?

____

____

____

____

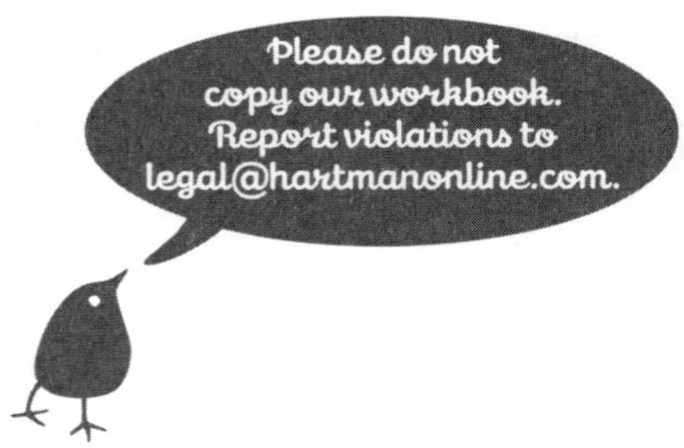

11

Human Development and Aging

1. Describe the stages of human development and identify common disorders for each group

True or False

1. ____ From the time an infant is born, it takes approximately 3 years for him to be able to move around, communicate basic needs, and feed himself.
2. ____ Infants develop from the hands to the head.
3. ____ HHAs should encourage infants to stand as soon as they can hold their heads up.
4. ____ Putting an infant to sleep on its back can reduce the risk of sudden infant death syndrome (SIDS).
5. ____ Tantrums are common among toddlers.
6. ____ The best way to deal with tantrums is to give the toddler what he wants.
7. ____ Preschool children are too young to know right from wrong.
8. ____ Children develop language skills between the ages of 3 and 5.
9. ____ From the ages of 5 to 10 years, children learn to get along with one another.
10. ____ School-age children (ages 5 to 10) develop cognitively and socially.
11. ____ Preadolescents are often easy to get along with and are able to handle more responsibility than younger children.
12. ____ Puberty is the stage of growth when secondary sex characteristics, such as body hair, appear.
13. ____ Most adolescents do not feel that peer acceptance is important.
14. ____ Adolescents may be moody due to changing hormones and body image concerns.
15. ____ Eating disorders are difficult to deal with but cannot be life-threatening.
16. ____ Due to changes they are experiencing, adolescents may become depressed and may attempt suicide.
17. ____ By 19 years of age, most young adults have stopped developing physically, psychologically, and socially.
18. ____ One developmental task that most young adults undertake is to choose an occupation or career.
19. ____ Middle-aged adults usually do not experience any physical changes due to aging.
20. ____ By the time a person reaches late adulthood, he is no longer able to develop new interests or make new friends.

2. Distinguish between fact (what is true) and fallacy (what is not true) about the aging process

True or False

1. ____ Older adults have different capabilities depending upon their health.

2. ____ As people age, they often become lonely, forgetful, and slow.

3. ____ Diseases and illnesses are not a normal part of aging.

4. ____ Many older adults can lead active and healthy lives.

5. ____ Prejudice against older people is as unfounded and unfair as prejudice against racial, ethnic, or religious groups.

6. ____ Movies often present an accurate image of what it is like to grow old.

3. Discuss normal changes of aging and list care guidelines

Multiple Choice

1. Older adults experience changes in their skin due to aging because
   (A) Much of the fatty layer beneath the skin is lost
   (B) They develop allergies to skin care products
   (C) Circulation to the skin is increased
   (D) There is not enough moisture in the air

2. Normal changes of aging in the musculoskeletal system include
   (A) Brittle bones
   (B) More flexible joints
   (C) Stronger muscles
   (D) Increased appetite

3. For clients who have poor vision, the HHA should
   (A) Discourage wearing sunglasses outside
   (B) Keep eyeglasses clean
   (C) Dim the lights
   (D) Have them read a newspaper daily

4. For clients who have trouble hearing, the HHA should
   (A) Speak in a low-pitched voice
   (B) Exaggerate her movements as she speaks
   (C) Shout to be heard
   (D) Remove excess earwax if possible

5. For clients with a decreased sense of taste and smell, the HHA should
   (A) Stop seasoning foods
   (B) Make sure there are working smoke detectors in the home
   (C) Only cook spicy meals
   (D) Perform oral care less often

6. For clients who have a decreased sense of touch, the HHA should
   (A) Serve food at hotter temperatures
   (B) Bathe these clients less often
   (C) Keep heating pads on the skin longer
   (D) Be careful when serving hot drinks

7. Clients with heart conditions should
   (A) Exercise vigorously to regain strength
   (B) Avoid vigorous activity
   (C) Avoid doing any activity
   (D) Stand up quickly to avoid dizziness

8. If a client is cold due to poor circulation, the best response by the HHA is to
   (A) Use a heating pad on the client's legs and arms
   (B) Remove the client's slippers
   (C) Layer the client's clothing
   (D) Put a hot water bottle on the client's feet

9. The best position for clients who have difficulty breathing is usually
   (A) Lying on the left side
   (B) Lying on the stomach
   (C) Lying flat on the back
   (D) Sitting upright

10. Older clients may need to urinate more frequently due to
    (A) The bladder not being able to hold as much urine
    (B) Drinking more fluids than younger adults
    (C) Incontinence
    (D) Being thirsty more often

11. Which of the following statements is true of urinary incontinence?
    (A) It is a normal part of getting older.
    (B) It could be a sign of illness.
    (C) It occurs when a person drinks too much fluid.
    (D) It is treated by withholding fluids.

12. Constipation could be the result of
    (A) Faster digestion process due to aging
    (B) Eating too much food during the day
    (C) Getting too much fiber in the diet
    (D) Slower peristalsis

13. Because insulin production lessens due to aging, some clients may
    (A) Need to take insulin to regulate blood sugar
    (B) Need to fast each day
    (C) Eat more sugary foods to increase insulin levels
    (D) Have the HHA give hormone injections

14. Normal changes in the reproductive system due to aging often result in
    (A) Loss of sexual drive
    (B) Thinning of vaginal walls in females
    (C) Inappropriate sexual advances
    (D) Decrease in the size of the prostate gland in males

15. Which of the following is a result of a weakened immune system due to normal changes of aging?
    (A) Increased risk of infection
    (B) More bouts of insomnia
    (C) Lower risk of falls
    (D) Increased risk of hypertension

16. Insomnia, withdrawal, and moodiness are common signs of
    (A) Anorexia
    (B) Depression
    (C) Confusion
    (D) Forgetfulness

17. Which of the following is a healthy way for an HHA to respond to a client's lifestyle changes due to aging?
    (A) Assume that the client is depressed and needs medication
    (B) Insist that the client discuss her feelings
    (C) Listen to the client if she wants to discuss her feelings
    (D) Talk about the HHA's own problems to make the client forget her problems

18. What is the most important thing for an HHA to do if she observes any changes in her client's condition?
    (A) Ask the family if they have seen the same changes
    (B) Call a spiritual leader of the client's choosing
    (C) Call the client's primary care provider
    (D) Report it to her supervisor

4. Identify attitudes and habits that promote health

Short Answer

List six things that HHAs can do to encourage clients to stay active, maintain self-esteem, and live independently.

____

____

____

____

____

____

____

____

____

Name: ____________________

Please do not
copy our workbook.
Report violations to
legal@hartmanonline.com.

12

Positioning, Transfers, and Ambulation

1. Explain positioning and describe how to safely position clients

Labeling

Label each position illustrated below and describe appropriate comfort measures for each.

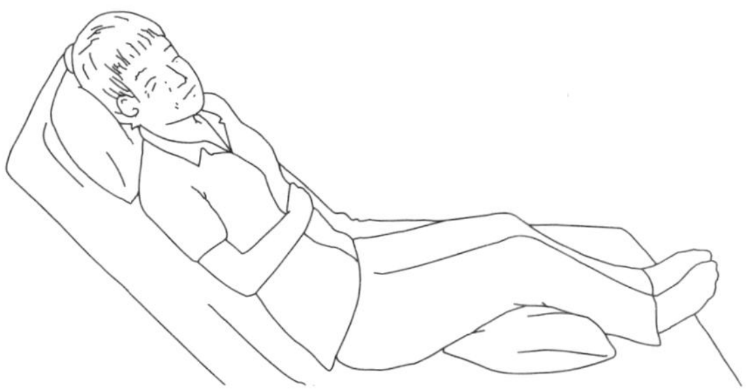

1. ______________________

Comfort measures: ______________________

____

____

____

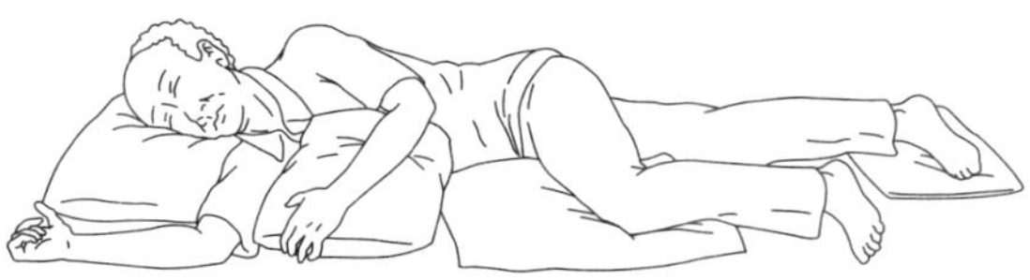

2. ______________________

Comfort measures: ______________________

____

____

____

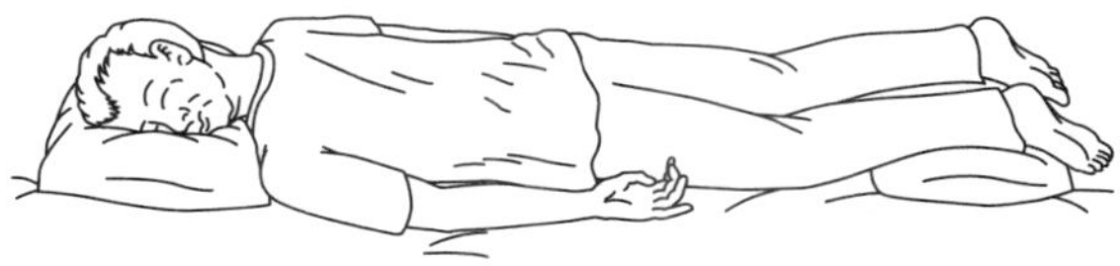

3. ______________________

Comfort measures: ______________________

____

____

____

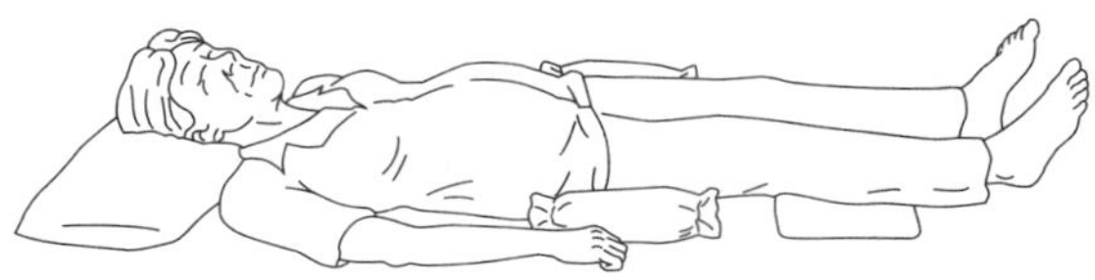

4. ______________________

Comfort measures: ______________________

____

____

____

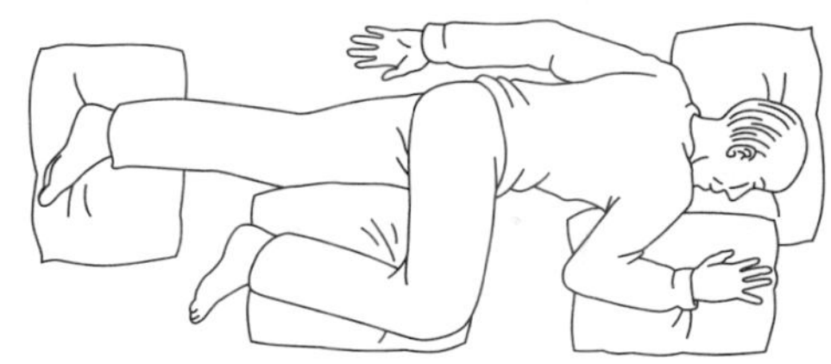

5. ______________________

Comfort measures: ______________________

____

____

____

Multiple Choice

6. How often do clients in wheelchairs need to be repositioned?
   (A) Once every hour
   (B) Once every 3 hours
   (C) Once per shift
   (D) Once before the HHA leaves the home

7. In this position, the client is lying on either side:
   (A) Supine
   (B) Lateral
   (C) Prone
   (D) Fowler

8. In this position, the client is lying on his stomach:
   (A) Sims
   (B) Lateral
   (C) Prone
   (D) Fowler

9. Logrolling is
   (A) A way to measure a bedbound client's weight
   (B) One way to record vital signs for clients who cannot get out of bed easily
   (C) Moving a client as a unit without disturbing alignment
   (D) A special method of bedmaking

10. Dangling is
    (A) Lying in the supine position
    (B) Doing a few sit-ups in bed to get used to the upright position
    (C) Elevating the client's feet with pillows
    (D) A way to help clients regain balance before standing up

11. A client in the Fowler position is
    (A) In a semisitting position (45 to 60 degrees)
    (B) Lying flat on their back
    (C) In a left side-lying position
    (D) Lying on their stomach

12. A draw sheet is used to
    (A) Make changing the bottom bed sheet easier
    (B) Help clients sleep better
    (C) Reposition clients without causing shearing
    (D) Clean up after episodes of incontinence

2. Describe how to safely transfer clients

Multiple Choice

1. Which of the following is an accurate guideline for HHAs working with clients in wheelchairs?
   (A) Before transferring a client, the HHA should make sure the wheelchair is unlocked and movable.
   (B) The HHA should check the client's alignment in the chair after a transfer is complete.
   (C) To fold a standard wheelchair, the HHA should turn it upside down to make the seat flatten.
   (D) All clients will need their HHA to transfer them to their wheelchairs.

2. Some clients have a side of the body that is weaker than the other one. The weaker side of the body should be referred to as the
   (A) Released side
   (B) Separated side
   (C) Ambulated side
   (D) Involved side

3. When applying a transfer belt, the HHA should place it
   (A) Around the wheelchair's backrest
   (B) Underneath the client's clothing, on bare skin
   (C) Over the client's clothing and around the waist
   (D) Around the HHA's waist so the client can hold on to it

4. The following piece of equipment may be used to help transfer a client who is unable to bear weight on her legs:
   (A) Sling
   (B) Slide board
   (C) Wheeled table
   (D) Folded blanket

5. Which of the following statements is true of using mechanical (hydraulic) lifts to assist with transfers?
   (A) When doing this type of transfer, it is safer for one person to transfer the client by himself.
   (B) The legs of the stand need to be closed, in their narrowest position, before helping the client into the lift.
   (C) Lifts help prevent injury to the HHA and the client.
   (D) It is best to use mechanical lifts when moving the client a long distance.

6. When transferring clients who have a one-sided weakness, which side moves first?
   (A) Left side
   (B) Either side
   (C) Weaker side
   (D) Stronger side

3. Discuss how to safely ambulate a client

Multiple Choice

1. If a client starts to fall while walking, the best response by the HHA would be to
   (A) Widen his stance and bring the client's body close to him
   (B) Catch the client under the arms to stop the fall
   (C) Move out of the way to allow the client to fall because the HHA could be injured trying to break the fall
   (D) Let the client fall on top of the HHA to break the fall

2. If a client falls, what is the first thing the HHA should do?
   (A) Help the client get up and into bed
   (B) Help the client walk around the room until she is steady
   (C) Call for help
   (D) Give the client ibuprofen and perform a physical examination to check for broken bones

3. A client who has some difficulty with balance but can bear weight on both legs should use a
   (A) Walker
   (B) Crutch
   (C) Wheelchair
   (D) Transfer board

4. Ambulation is another word for
   (A) Moving or walking
   (B) Positioning
   (C) Transferring
   (D) Logrolling

5. In addition to a transfer belt, what equipment should the HHA have when assisting a client to ambulate?
   (A) Mechanical lift
   (B) Rocking chair
   (C) Extra pillows
   (D) Nonskid shoes

6. If the client is unable to stand without help, the HHA should
   (A) Hold the client close to the HHA's center of gravity
   (B) Tell the client to stand on the count of 3
   (C) Brace the client's lower extremities
   (D) Adjust the bed to its highest position

7. When helping a client who is visually impaired to walk, it is important for the HHA to
   (A) Keep the client in front of her
   (B) Be beside and slightly ahead of the client
   (C) Walk quickly
   (D) Avoid mentioning stepping up or down

Name: ____________________

8. Which of the following assistive devices for walking has four rubber-tipped feet?
   (A) C cane
   (B) Quad cane
   (C) Crutch
   (D) Transfer belt

9. When using a cane, the client should place it on their ________ side.
   (A) Left
   (B) Right
   (C) Weaker
   (D) Stronger

4. List ways to make clients more comfortable

Short Answer

1. List four things the HHA can do to provide for the comfort and safety of clients in and around the bed.

____

____

____

____

____

____

____

____

____

____

____

2. Name two benefits of giving a client a back massage.

____

____

____

____

____

____

____

____

____

Matching

Use each letter only once.

3. ____ Abduction pillows
4. ____ Backrests
5. ____ Bed cradles
6. ____ Bed tables
7. ____ Draw sheets
8. ____ Footboards
9. ____ Handrolls
10. ____ Orthotic devices
11. ____ Trochanter rolls

(A) Placed against the feet to keep them properly aligned and to prevent foot drop

(B) Keep bed covers from resting on the legs and feet

(C) Used to help clients who cannot help with turning or moving up in bed; help prevent skin damage from shearing

(D) Keep the hand and/or fingers in a normal, natural position

(E) Rolled towels or blankets that keep the hips and legs from turning outward

(F) Help support and align a limb and improve its functioning (e.g., a splint)

(G) Made of pillows, cardboard, or wood, they provide support for the back

(H) Keep food or other often-used items close to the client while he is in bed; one option can be made at home using a cardboard box

(I) Special pillows used to keep the hips in the proper position after hip surgery

13
Personal Care Skills

1. Describe the home health aide's role in assisting clients with personal care

Short Answer

1. Why should the HHA explain to the client what he will be doing before beginning a task?

____

____

____

____

2. List three things that the HHA should observe when providing or assisting with personal care.

____

____

____

____

2. Explain guidelines for assisting with bathing

True or False

1. ____ Bathing promotes health and removes perspiration and dirt from the skin.
2. ____ The axillae (underarms) should be washed 3 times per week.
3. ____ When washing a client's eyes and face, the HHA should use a warm, soapy washcloth.
4. ____ The perineum should be washed every day.
5. ____ Older skin produces more perspiration than younger skin.
6. ____ The client should test the temperature of the water before bathing because she is best able to choose a comfortable water temperature.
7. ____ When washing a female's perineal area, the HHA should wipe from back to front.
8. ____ Using bath oils during baths is helpful for clients with dry skin.
9. ____ Checking to make sure the room is warm enough for the client before bathing is important.
10. ____ Before performing perineal care, the HHA should change his gloves.
11. ____ Clients who have textured hair need their hair washed more often than clients with straight hair.

3. Describe guidelines for assisting with grooming

Complete the Sentence

1. It is better for a client to wear *pajamas* | *regular clothes* during the day.
2. The *HHA* | *client* should choose a client's clothing for the day.
3. *Front-fastening* | *back-fastening* bras are easier for clients to work for themselves.
4. When dressing a client who has weakness or paralysis on one side, the HHA should dress the *weaker* | *stronger* side first.
5. Clothing that is *smaller* | *larger* than the client normally wears is easier to put on.

6. If a client has no cuts on his face, the HHA *should still* | *does not need to* wear gloves while shaving him.
7. Lice eggs are *black and powdery* | *brown or white*.
8. When providing foot care, the HHA *should* | *should not* put lotion on dry areas between the toes.
9. When assisting with grooming, the HHA should *let the client do all he can for himself* | *do as much as possible for the client*.
10. Before giving nail care to a client, the HHA should *soak* | *scrub* the client's hands and nails for at least 5 minutes.
11. Clients who are taking anticoagulant medication (blood thinners) should be shaved with a(n) *electric* | *safety* razor.

4. Identify guidelines for oral care

Multiple Choice

1. When must oral care be done?
   (A) After the last meal or snack of the day
   (B) Before lunch is eaten
   (C) After the afternoon snack
   (D) Before dinner is served
2. The inhalation of food, fluid, or foreign material into the lungs is called
   (A) Peristalsis
   (B) Aspiration
   (C) Pediculosis
   (D) Hygiene
3. In which position should an unconscious client be placed before giving oral care?
   (A) Sitting upright
   (B) Flat on their back
   (C) Reclining slightly in a chair
   (D) Turned on their side
4. Dentures must be handled carefully because
   (A) A client may not be able to eat without them
   (B) They do not cost much
   (C) A client will look unattractive without them
   (D) They are sharp
5. How should dentures be stored?
   (A) In denture solution
   (B) On the counter near the sink
   (C) Wrapped in a paper towel
   (D) In hot water
6. If an HHA is reinserting a client's dentures, the client should be
   (A) Lying flat on his back
   (B) Standing
   (C) Sitting upright
   (D) Lying down on his side

5. Explain care guidelines for prosthetic devices

True or False

1. ____ Hearing aids should be soaked in warm water before cleaning them.
2. ____ When cleaning the eyelid after an artificial eye is removed, the HHA should wipe gently from the outer area toward the inner area.
3. ____ Prostheses are relatively inexpensive and are easy to replace.
4. ____ Artificial eyes are held in place by a special type of glue.
5. ____ In general, hearing aids should be cleaned daily.
6. ____ A prosthesis is a device that replaces a body part that is missing or deformed because of an accident, injury, illness, or birth defect.
7. ____ Artificial eyes should be rinsed in rubbing alcohol to prevent infection.
8. ____ If a prosthesis is broken, it is best for the HHA to try to repair it before bothering her supervisor about it.
9. ____ When observing the skin on the stump, it is important that the HHA check for signs of skin breakdown.

6. Explain guidelines for assisting with elimination

Multiple Choice

1. A fracture pan is used for urination with
   (A) Any client who cannot get out of bed
   (B) Clients who cannot raise their hips
   (C) Clients who have problems with incontinence
   (D) Clients who have difficulty urinating

2. Men will generally use a ____________ for urination when they cannot get out of bed.
   (A) Urinal
   (B) Fracture pan
   (C) Toilet
   (D) Portable commode

3. Clients who can get out of bed but cannot walk to the bathroom may use a(n)
   (A) Toilet
   (B) Urinal
   (C) Portable commode
   (D) Indwelling catheter

4. The best position for bowel elimination is
   (A) Squatting and leaning forward
   (B) Lying flat on the back
   (C) Lying on the left side
   (D) Leaning backward

5. Which of the following statements is true of properly positioning a standard bedpan?
   (A) A standard bedpan should be positioned with the narrower end aligned with the client's buttocks.
   (B) A standard bedpan can be positioned either toward the foot or head of the bed.
   (C) A standard bedpan should be positioned with the wider end aligned with the client's buttocks.
   (D) A standard bedpan should be positioned sideways and slightly tilted.

6. When should the removable container in a portable commode be cleaned?
   (A) After each use
   (B) Once a week
   (C) When the client requests it to be cleaned
   (D) Once per hour

7. Describe how to dispose of body wastes

Short Answer

1. How must washcloths that have been used to clean perineal areas be washed?

____

____

____

____

2. Why must gloves be worn when handling bedpans, urinals, or basins that contain wastes?

____

____

____

____

Name: ______________________________

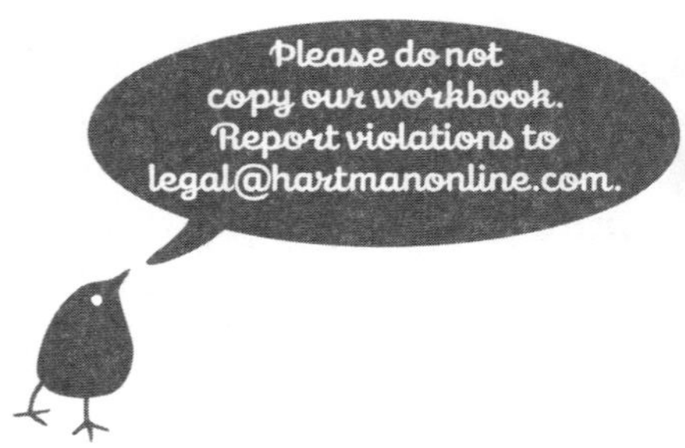
Please do not
copy our workbook.
Report violations to
legal@hartmanonline.com.

14

Core Healthcare Skills

1. Explain the importance of monitoring vital signs

Short Answer

1. What may changes in vital signs indicate?

____

____

____

____

2. Which changes should be immediately reported to a supervisor?

____

____

____

____

____

____

3. What are five sites for measuring body temperature?

____

____

____

____

____

____

Short Answer

Mark an X by each person for whom an oral temperature should NOT be taken.

4. ____ Person is disoriented.
5. ____ Person has sores in his mouth.
6. ____ Person is 40 years old.
7. ____ Person is unconscious.
8. ____ Person has a broken leg.
9. ____ Person is likely to have a seizure.
10. ____ Person has facial paralysis.
11. ____ Person has had children.

Short Answer

For each of the illustrations of thermometers shown below, write the temperature reading to the nearest tenth (0.1) degree in the blank provided.

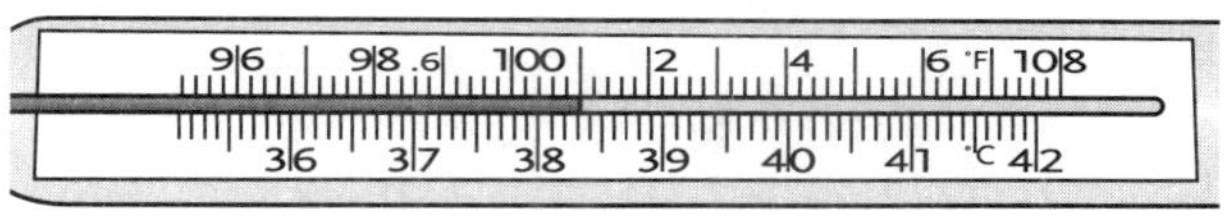

12. ______________________

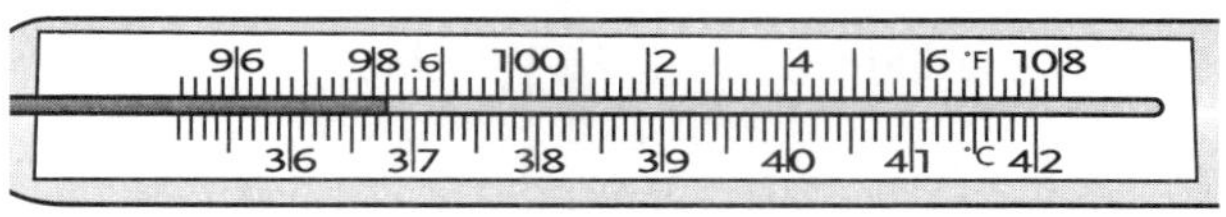

13. ______________________

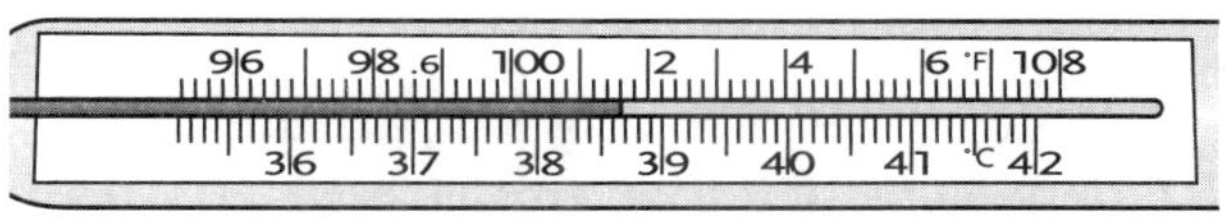

14. ______________________

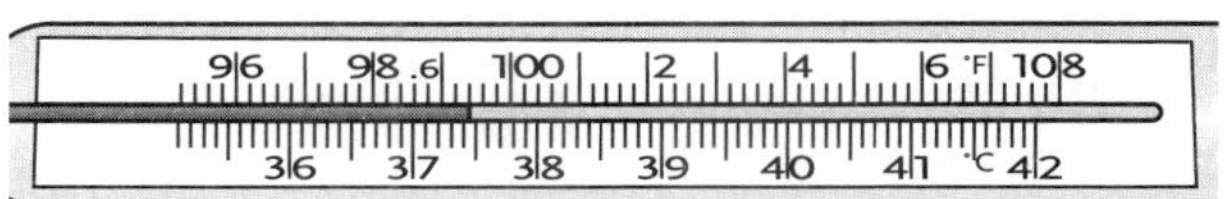

15. ______________________

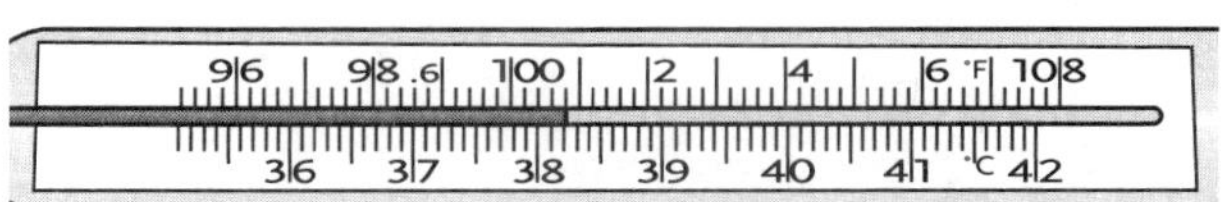

16. ______________________

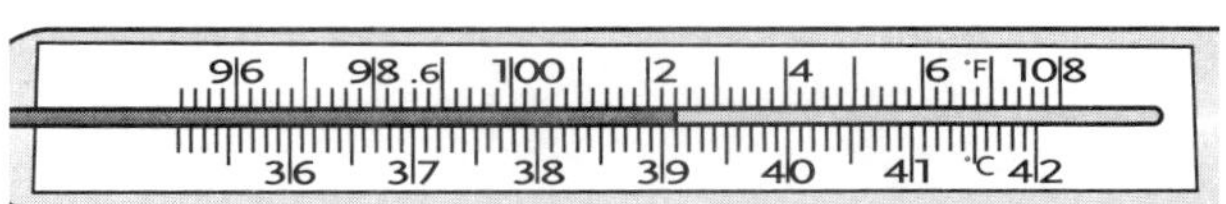

17. ______________________

Name: ____________________

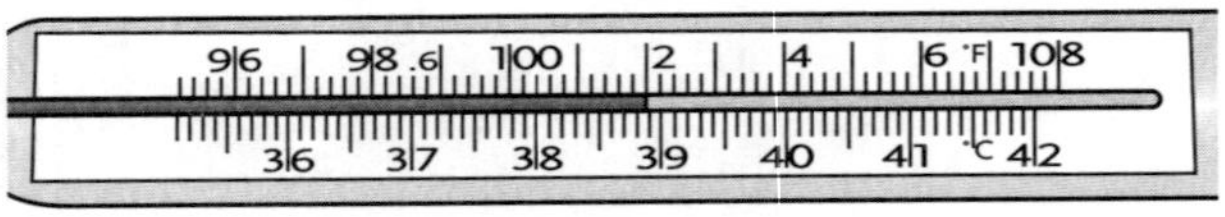

18. ____________________

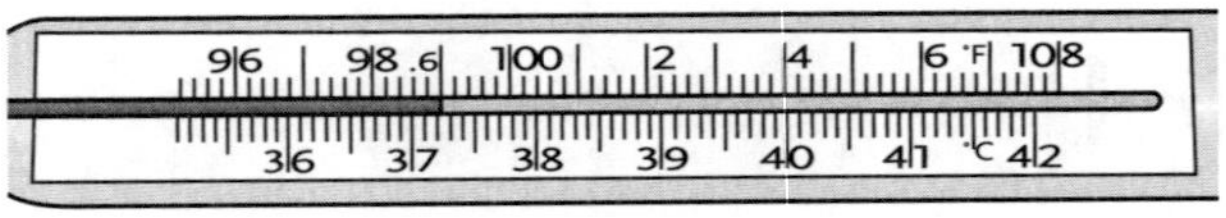

19. ____________________

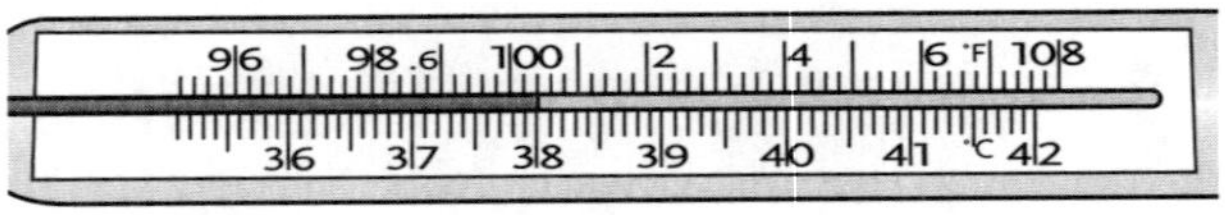

20. ____________________

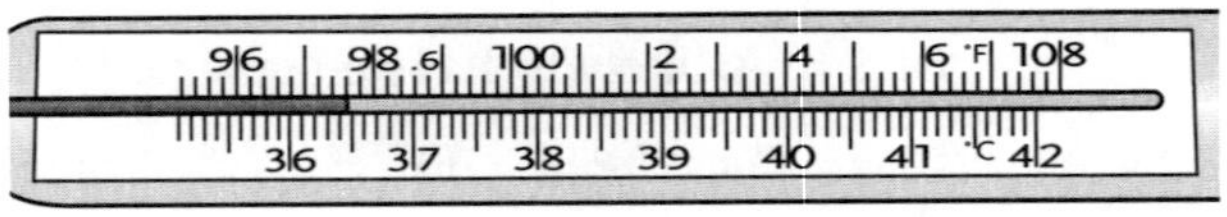

21. ____________________

Multiple Choice

22. Which of the following is the normal temperature range for the oral method?
    (A) 90.6–94.6 degrees Fahrenheit
    (B) 93.6–97.9 degrees Fahrenheit
    (C) 98.6–100.6 degrees Fahrenheit
    (D) 97.6–99.6 degrees Fahrenheit

23. Which of the following thermometers is used to take a temperature in the ear?
    (A) Temporal artery thermometer
    (B) Rectal thermometer
    (C) Axillary thermometer
    (D) Tympanic thermometer

24. Which of the following temperature sites is another word for the armpit area?
    (A) Temporal artery
    (B) Rectum
    (C) Axilla
    (D) Tympanum

25. Which temperature site is considered to be the most accurate?
    (A) Mouth (oral)
    (B) Rectum (rectal)
    (C) Temporal artery (forehead)
    (D) Ear (tympanic)

26. A rectal thermometer is usually color-coded
    (A) Red
    (B) Green
    (C) Black
    (D) Blue

27. What is the most common site for monitoring the pulse rate?
    (A) Apical pulse
    (B) Femoral pulse
    (C) Pedal pulse
    (D) Radial pulse

28. For adults, the normal pulse rate is
    (A) 20 to 40 beats per minute
    (B) 40 to 60 beats per minute
    (C) 60 to 100 beats per minute
    (D) 90 to 120 beats per minute

29. The medical term for rapid pulse rate is
    (A) Bradypnea
    (B) Bradycardia
    (C) Tachypnea
    (D) Tachycardia

30. The medical term for difficulty breathing is
    (A) Dyspeptic
    (B) Dyspnea
    (C) Dysphagia
    (D) Dystolic

31. The medical term for rapid respirations is
    (A) Apnea
    (B) Eupnea
    (C) Orthopnea
    (D) Tachypnea

32. The normal respiration rate for adults ranges from
    (A) 5 to 10 breaths per minute
    (B) 7 to 11 breaths per minute
    (C) 12 to 20 breaths per minute
    (D) 25 to 32 breaths per minute

33. Why is it important for the HHA to observe respirations without letting the client know what she is doing?
    (A) People may breathe more quickly if they know they are being observed.
    (B) People will hold their breath if they know what the HHA wants to measure.
    (C) The procedure takes less time if the client is unaware of what is happening.
    (D) Observing respirations is a painful process for most people.

34. Which of the following is considered an *elevated* blood pressure reading?
    (A) 120/70
    (B) 130/75
    (C) 110/70
    (D) 100/79

35. Which of the following is used to measure blood pressure?
    (A) Sphygmomanometer
    (B) Urostoscope
    (C) Reflex hammer
    (D) Otoscope

36. The second measurement of blood pressure reflects the phase when the heart relaxes. It is called the __________ phase.
    (A) Systolic
    (B) Mercurial
    (C) Hyperbolic
    (D) Diastolic

37. Blood pressure measurements are recorded as
    (A) Rhythms
    (B) Fractions
    (C) Decimals
    (D) Equations

38. Which measurement of blood pressure is always higher than the other?
    (A) Systolic
    (B) Dystemic
    (C) Diastolic
    (D) Systemic

Short Answer

For each of the gauges shown below, record the blood pressure shown and answer the question.

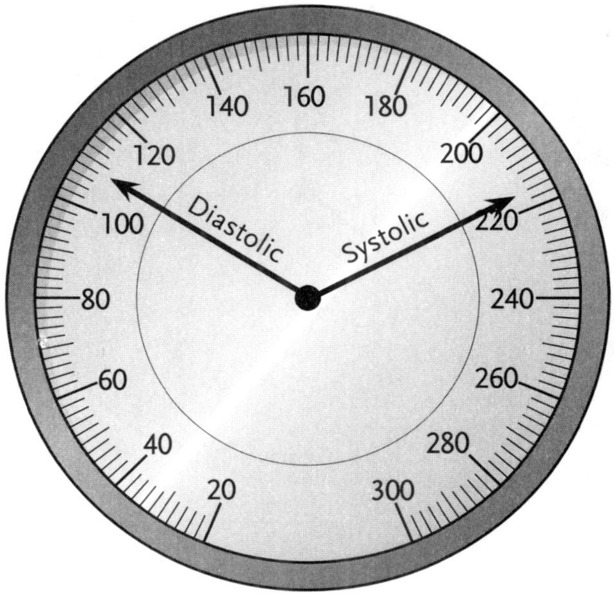

39. ______________________________

Is this reading within normal range?

____

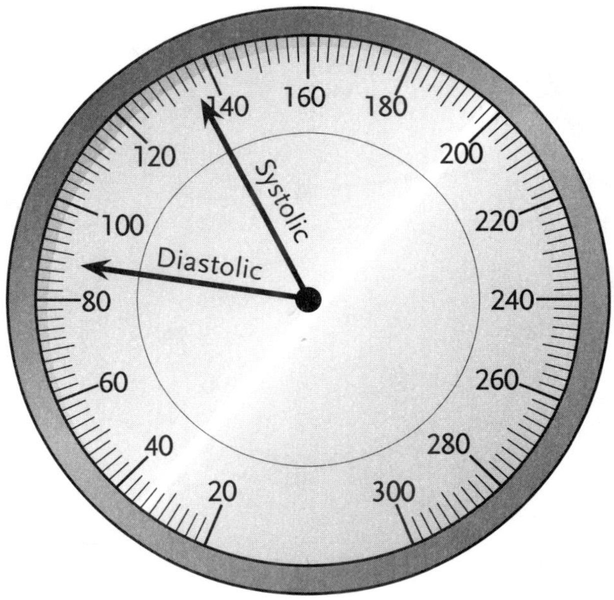

40. ______________________________

Is this reading within normal range?

____

Name: ______________________

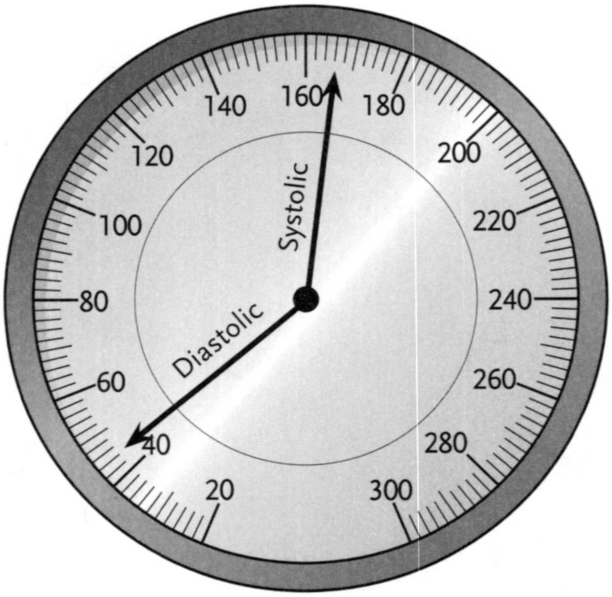

41. ______________________

Is this reading within normal range?

____

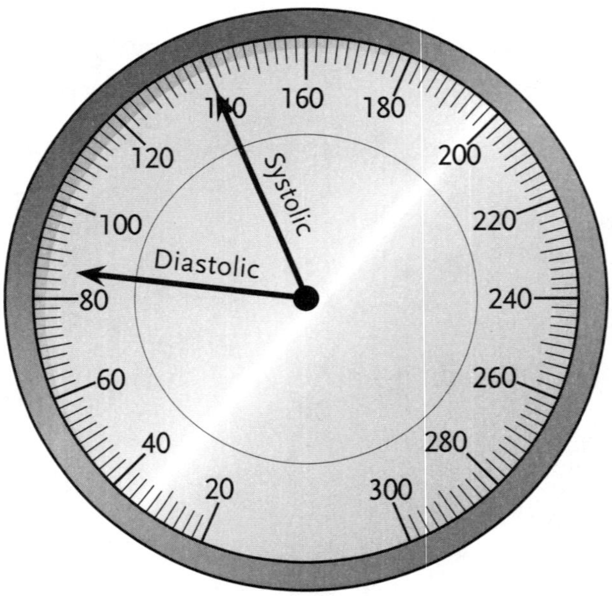

42. ______________________

Is this reading within normal range?

____

Short Answer

43. If a client complains of pain, what questions should the HHA ask to get the most accurate information?

____

____

____

____

____

____

____

____

____

____

____

Short Answer

Looking at each of the readings shown below, determine each client's weight for questions 44 to 47 and height for questions 48 to 51.

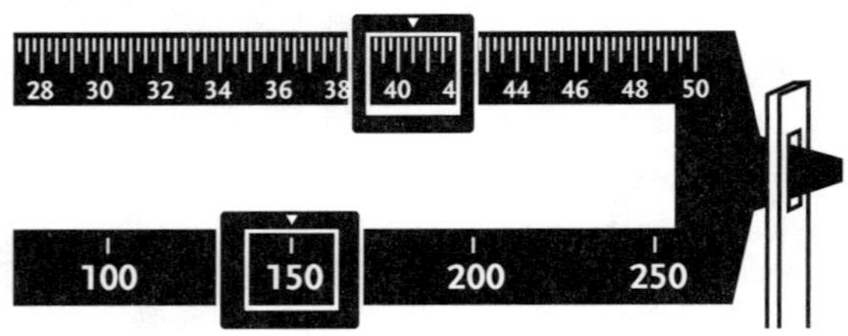

44. ______________________

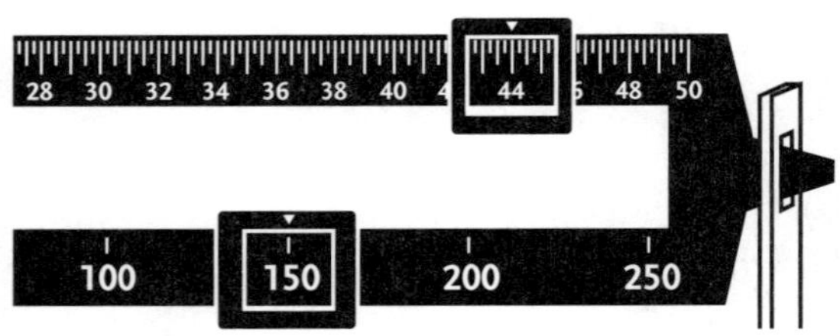

45. ______________________

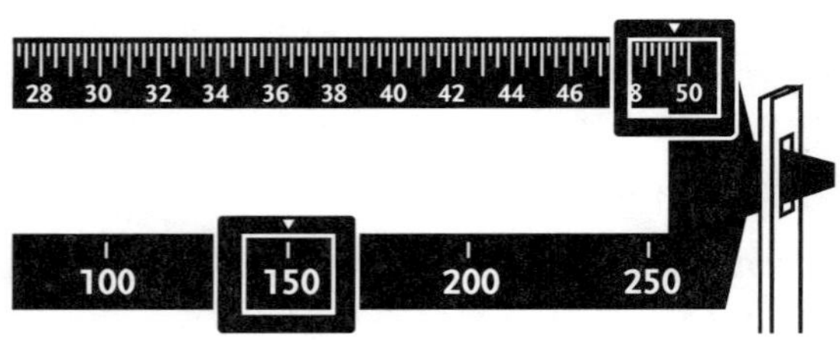

46. ______________________

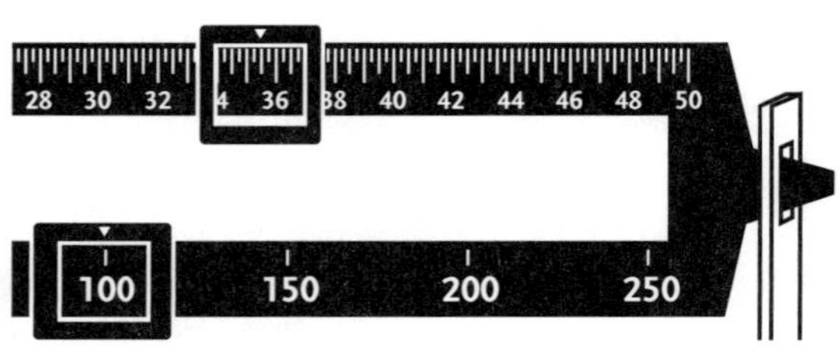

47. ______________________

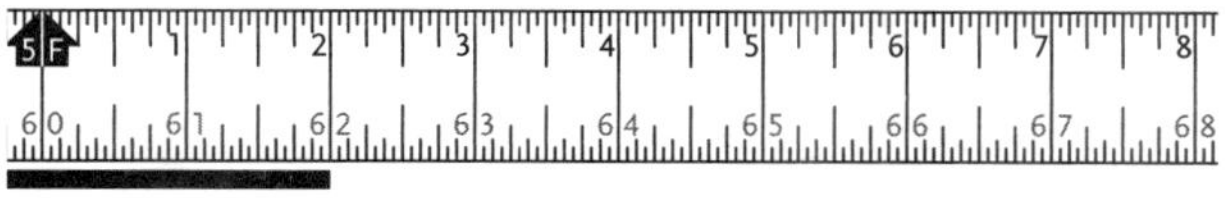

48. ______________________

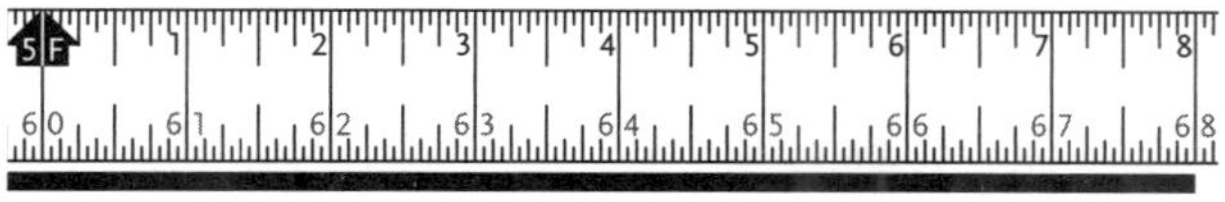

49. ______________________

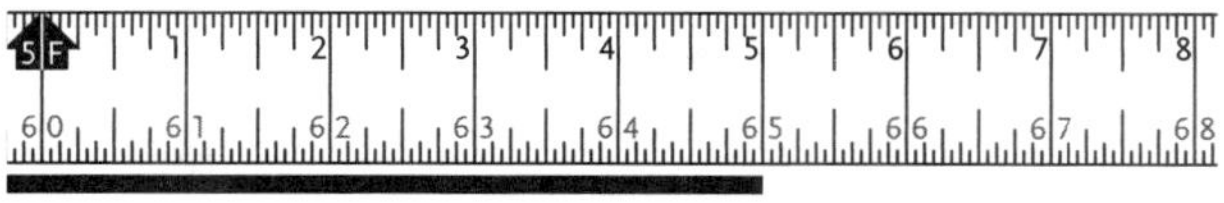

50. ______________________

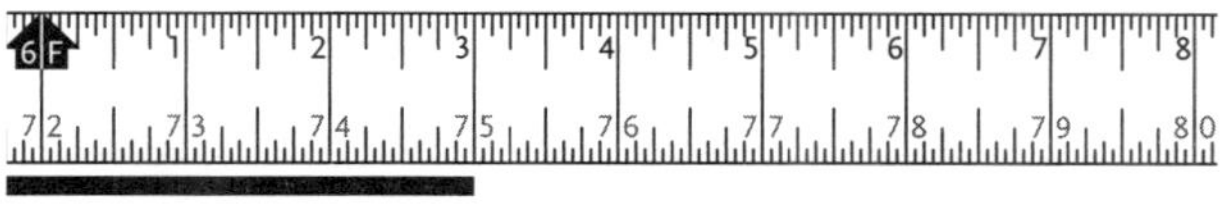

51. ______________________

2. List three types of specimens that may be collected from a client

Matching

Use each letter only once.

1. _____ 24-hour urine specimen
2. _____ Clean-catch specimen
3. _____ Hat
4. _____ Routine urine specimen
5. _____ Specimen
6. _____ Sputum specimen
7. _____ Stool specimen

(A) Collection container put into the toilet bowl to collect and measure stool and urine

(B) Urine and toilet paper should not be included with this specimen

(C) A sample that is used for analysis in order to try to make a diagnosis

(D) Urine sample collected any time the client voids

(E) Excludes the first and last urine voided from the sample

(F) A specimen used to test for certain chemicals and hormones that usually begins at 7 a.m. and ends at 7 a.m. the following day

(G) A specimen of thick mucus that is best collected in the early morning

3. Describe the importance of fluid balance and explain intake and output (I&O)

True or False

1. _____ Fluids come in the form of liquids a person drinks, as well as semiliquid foods such as soup or gelatin.
2. _____ The fluid a person consumes is called *intake* or *input.*
3. _____ All the body's fluid output is in the form of urine.
4. _____ Fluid balance means taking in and eliminating equal amounts of fluid.
5. _____ Most people need to consciously monitor their fluid balance.

Conversions

6. Mrs. Wyant drinks half of a glass of orange juice. The glass holds about 1 cup of liquid.

   How many milliliters of orange juice did Mrs. Wyant drink?

   ______________________ mL

7. Mr. Ramirez just ate some chocolate pudding from a 6-ounce container. The leftover pudding is measured and is about 35 mL.

   How many milliliters of pudding did Mr. Ramirez eat?

   ______________________ mL

8. Ms. Sumiko has a bowl of soup for lunch. The soup bowl holds about 1½ cups of liquid.

   How many milliliters is this?

   ______________________ mL

   Ms. Sumiko finishes most of her soup, but leaves about 25 mL.

   How many mL of soup did Ms. Sumiko eat?

   ______________________ mL

Name: ____________________

Short Answer

9. List three guidelines that an HHA should follow when a client vomits.

____

____

____

____

____

____

____

4. Describe guidelines for catheter care

Matching

Use each letter only once.

1. ____ Catheter
2. ____ Condom catheter
3. ____ Indwelling catheter
4. ____ Straight catheter
5. ____ Urinary catheter

(A) Urinary catheter that has an attachment that fits onto the penis

(B) Urinary catheter that is removed immediately after urine is drained

(C) Thin tube used to drain urine from the bladder

(D) Urinary catheter that remains inside the bladder for a period of time

(E) Thin tube inserted into the body that is used to drain or inject fluids

True or False

6. ____ The drainage bag for a urinary catheter must always be kept lower than the bladder or hips.

7. ____ For clients who have urinary catheters, daily care of the genital area is important to avoid infection.

8. ____ The HHA is responsible for removing a urinary catheter once the doctor says it is no longer needed.

9. ____ When cleaning the area near the catheter, the HHA should use a clean area of the washcloth for each stroke and move away from the meatus.

5. Explain the benefits of warm and cold applications

Crossword

Across

3. Cold applications can bring this down.
4. Type of application that helps stop bleeding
6. A warm soak of the perineal area to clean perineal wounds and reduce pain

Down

1. A condition that could cause a person to be unable to feel or notice damage occurring from a warm or cold application
2. This type of pack is a cold application HHAs may be allowed to prepare and apply.
5. Type of application that increases blood flow to an injured area

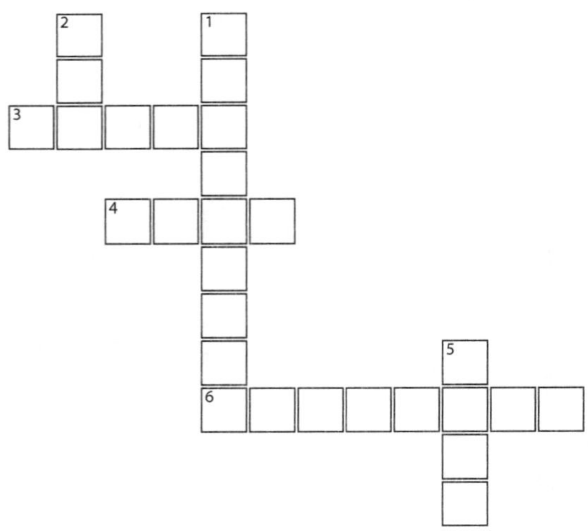

Multiple Choice

7. Which of the following is a type of dry warm application?
   (A) Cold compress
   (B) Warm tub bath
   (C) Warm soak
   (D) Disposable warm pack

8. A benefit of heat is that it
   (A) Increases blood flow to the affected area
   (B) Decreases oxygen to the tissues
   (C) Brings down high fevers
   (D) Causes numbness in the affected area

9. Which of the following is a type of moist cold application?
   (A) Sitz bath
   (B) Warm compress
   (C) Disposable cold pack
   (D) Ice pack

10. What is the proper water temperature when making a warm compress?
   (A) No higher than 95 degrees Fahrenheit
   (B) No higher than 105 degrees Fahrenheit
   (C) No higher than 120 degrees Fahrenheit
   (D) No higher than 125 degrees Fahrenheit

6. Explain how to apply nonsterile dressings

Short Answer

What is the difference between sterile and nonsterile dressings?

____

____

____

____

____

____

____

____

7. Describe the purpose of compression stockings and how to apply them

Multiple Choice

1. Why are compression stockings ordered for some clients?
   (A) They help prevent diabetes.
   (B) They help prevent anemia.
   (C) They help prevent swelling and promote blood circulation.
   (D) They help prevent chronic obstructive pulmonary disease.

2. The best time to apply compression stockings is
   (A) In the evening, before the client goes to bed
   (B) In the morning, before the client gets out of bed
   (C) In the early afternoon, before the client gets back in bed to rest
   (D) In the late morning, before the client has lunch

3. Where should the heel of the stocking be after the stocking is applied?
   (A) Over the client's toes
   (B) Over the client's heel
   (C) Over the client's lower calf
   (D) Over the client's shin

8. Define *ostomy* and list care guidelines

True or False

1. ____ An ostomy is the surgical creation of an opening from an area inside the body to the outside.

2. ____ The artificial opening in the abdomen through which stool is eliminated is called a *stoma*.

3. ____ Clients who have ileostomies will need to restrict their fluid intake.

4. ____ The HHA should wear gloves when providing ostomy care.

Name: ______________________________

Multiple Choice

5. Which of the following is part of providing professional ostomy care?
   (A) Telling clients to stop being embarrassed about having an ostomy
   (B) Using colorful nicknames to refer to the ostomy bag
   (C) Always providing privacy
   (D) Squinting while providing care to avoid looking at the ostomy

6. What could cause a food blockage in a client who has an ileostomy?
   (A) Too much liquid
   (B) A large amount of high-fiber food
   (C) Having an ostomy pouch that is ¼ full
   (D) Using skin barriers around the stoma

9. Describe how to assist with an elastic bandage

Multiple Choice

1. Elastic bandages are also known as
   (A) Nonsterile bandages
   (B) Plastic bandages
   (C) Liquid bandages
   (D) Aseptic bandages

2. One purpose of an elastic bandage is to
   (A) Elevate a cast
   (B) Hold a dressing in place
   (C) Cover a pressure injury
   (D) Help with ambulation

3. Elastic bandages should be applied snugly enough to control ________________ and prevent movement of ________________.
   (A) Temperature, the client
   (B) Bleeding, dressings
   (C) Elevation, dressings
   (D) Movement, the client

4. How soon should the HHA check on a client after applying a bandage?
   (A) 45 to 60 minutes
   (B) 30 to 40 minutes
   (C) 2 to 3 hours
   (D) 10 to 15 minutes

15
Medications and Technology in Home Care

1. List four guidelines for safe and proper use of medications

True or False

1. ____ HHAs must not handle or give medications unless specifically trained and assigned to do so.
2. ____ HHAs are not allowed to touch the client's medication containers in any way.
3. ____ It is not important for an HHA to know what medications the client is taking, as long as the HHA documents when they are taken.
4. ____ HHAs should report symptoms such as stomachache or vomiting because these could indicate a side effect or drug interaction.
5. ____ Aspirin is an example of an over-the-counter drug.

2. Identify the "rights" of medications

Multiple Choice

1. Checking the label for instructions on how the medication should be taken (how it enters the body) is which right of medication?
   (A) The right client
   (B) The right route
   (C) The right time
   (D) The right medication
2. Checking the label for instructions on how much medication to take is which right of medication?
   (A) The right dose
   (B) The right client
   (C) The right time
   (D) The right route
3. Making sure the medication name on the container matches the name listed in the care plan is which right of medication?
   (A) The right time
   (B) The right medication
   (C) The right client
   (D) The right dose
4. Recording that a client has taken a medication is which right of medication?
   (A) The right client
   (B) The right dose
   (C) The right time
   (D) The right documentation
5. Checking the label to make sure the client's name is on it is which right of medication?
   (A) The right client
   (B) The right medication
   (C) The right time
   (D) The right route
6. Checking the label for instructions on how often the medication should be taken is which right of medication?
   (A) The right route
   (B) The right client
   (C) The right time
   (D) The right dose

Name: ____________________

3. Explain how to assist a client with self-administered medications

Complete the Sentence

1. *All medications are | Some medications may be* taken with food to avoid stomach irritation.
2. To avoid any problems with drug interactions, the HHA should document every medication the client takes, *whether or not it is in the care plan | as long as it is in the care plan.*
3. Sedatives should never be mixed with *grapefruit juice | alcohol.*
4. The HHA *can | cannot* remind a client when it is time to take medication.
5. Allergic reactions to medication *do not | may* require emergency help.

Short Answer

6. List seven ways in which HHAs may help clients with self-medication.

7. List 10 actions involving self-medication that HHAs are NOT allowed to do.

8. Name five common side effects that clients may experience from their medications.

4. Identify observations about medications that should be reported right away

Short Answer

1. What should the HHA do if a client shows signs of a reaction to a medication or reports side effects?

____

____

____

2. What should the HHA do if a client takes the wrong dose, takes medication at the wrong time, or takes the wrong kind of medication?

____

____

____

5. Describe what to do in an emergency involving medications

Short Answer

1. Mrs. Mallory takes several prescription medications each day as ordered by her physician. One day her HHA arrives to find Mrs. Mallory sitting down in a chair and looking very ill. When the HHA asks her if she is okay, Mrs. Mallory says that she feels very sick to her stomach and thinks she might faint. Mrs. Mallory says that she might have taken too much medication because she could not remember if she had already taken her morning pill. What would be the best response by the HHA?

____

____

____

____

____

____

____

____

____

____

2. An HHA arrives at Mr. MacIntyre's home at 8:30 a.m. and finds him lying in bed. The HHA is unable to wake him, and then she notices several bottles of pills on the table next to the bed. They are all open, and some of the pills are scattered on the table and the floor. What would be the best response by the HHA?

____

____

____

____

____

____

____

____

____

____

____

6. Identify methods of medication storage

True or False

1. ____ The client's medication should be kept separate from medicine used by other members of the household.
2. ____ If young children are present in the home, medications should be stored on top of the counter.

3. ____ Medications should be stored away from heat and light.

4. ____ If a medication has expired, the HHA should discard it in the trash.

7. Identify signs of drug misuse and abuse and know how to report these

Multiple Choice

1. Proper medication usage includes which of the following?
   (A) Refusing to take medications
   (B) Taking medication with alcohol
   (C) Sharing medication with others
   (D) Taking the right dose at the right time

2. The best thing the HHA can do if a client refuses to take medication is to
   (A) Push the client to take the medication, explaining that it is good for him
   (B) Try to find out why the client does not want to take the medication and report to the supervisor
   (C) Call 911 for emergency medical help
   (D) Call the client's doctor immediately

3. A common reason why people avoid taking prescribed medication is
   (A) They dislike the side effects
   (B) They are stubborn
   (C) They do not want to feel better
   (D) They would rather get well without it

4. Signs of drug misuse or abuse include
   (A) Increased appetite and weight gain
   (B) Unusual cheerfulness
   (C) Depression and moodiness
   (D) Better relationships with family members

5. The drugs that pose the highest risk for causing drug dependency are
   (A) Pain medications
   (B) Antihistamines (allergy medicines)
   (C) Beta-blockers
   (D) Multivitamins

8. Demonstrate an understanding of oxygen equipment

True or False

1. ____ Oxygen therapy is the administration of oxygen to increase the supply of oxygen to the lungs.

2. ____ Oxygen is prescribed by a provider.

3. ____ HHAs are usually responsible for adjusting oxygen settings for clients.

4. ____ Oxygen supports combustion; this means it makes other things burn.

5. ____ A flammable liquid like alcohol can be kept near where oxygen is in use as long as it is covered.

6. ____ If oxygen is stored in a room but is not in use, the client can smoke in that room.

7. ____ Oxygen should be turned off in the event of a fire.

8. ____ It is important for the HHA to check the skin around oxygen masks and tubing for irritation.

9. ____ If a client has skin irritation around a nasal cannula, the HHA should use Vaseline to soften the skin.

Multiple Choice

10. Which of the following is a boxlike device that changes air in the room into air with more oxygen?
    (A) Oxygen cannula
    (B) Oxygen face mask
    (C) Oxygen concentrator
    (D) Oxygen prongs

11. Who is responsible for servicing oxygen tanks or concentrators in a client's home?
    (A) The provider who prescribed the oxygen
    (B) The HHA
    (C) The client's family members
    (D) The agency that supplies the oxygen

12. When should the HHA administer a client's oxygen?
    (A) Whenever the client requests that she do so
    (B) Every 3 days
    (C) According to the care plan
    (D) Never

13. Which of the following can liquid oxygen cause?
    (A) Frostbite
    (B) Addiction
    (C) Digestive problems
    (D) Heart failure

14. What kind of water is used in humidifying bottles for oxygen concentrators?
    (A) Sparkling water
    (B) Natural spring water
    (C) Distilled water
    (D) Tap water

15. What is the purpose of a humidifier?
    (A) To put only steam in the air
    (B) To remove moisture from the air
    (C) To put warm or cool moisture in the air
    (D) To filter the air

9. Explain care guidelines for intravenous (IV) therapy

Multiple Choice

1. IVs allow direct access to
   (A) The heart
   (B) The lungs
   (C) The bloodstream
   (D) The muscles

2. What is the HHA's responsibility for IV care?
   (A) Inserting IV lines
   (B) Removing IV lines
   (C) Care of the IV site
   (D) Documenting and reporting observations

3. Which of the following refers to treatments that are used in addition to the conventional treatments prescribed by a doctor?
   (A) Western medicine
   (B) Complementary medicine
   (C) Oxygen therapy
   (D) Respiratory medicine

4. Treating a person with acupuncture means
   (A) Putting the hands on both sides of the spine to realign it
   (B) Taking tablets that contain a specific healing substance
   (C) Using targeted laser light on specific body parts
   (D) Inserting very fine needles into points on the body

Name: ______________________________

16

Rehabilitation and Restorative Care

1. Discuss rehabilitation and restorative care

Short Answer

1. List four goals of a rehabilitative program.

____

____

____

____

____

____

____

2. What is the goal of restorative care?

____

____

____

2. Explain the home care rehabilitation model

Short Answer

List five members of the team who may participate in a client's restorative care.

____

____

____

____

____

____

3. Describe guidelines for assisting with rehabilitation and restorative care

True or False

1. ____ The HHA should ignore any setbacks a client experiences so the client does not become discouraged.
2. ____ All clients will enjoy being encouraged in an obvious way.
3. ____ The HHA should do everything for the client, rather than having him try to do it himself. Doing this will help speed recovery.
4. ____ The HHA should not report any decline in a client's ability because all clients in restorative care will have a decline in ability.
5. ____ Family members and clients will take cues from the HHA on how to behave.
6. ____ The HHA should break tasks down into small steps.
7. ____ It is important for the HHA to report any signs of depression or mood changes in a client.

4. Describe how to assist with range of motion exercises

Labeling

For the following illustrations, write the correct term for each body movement.

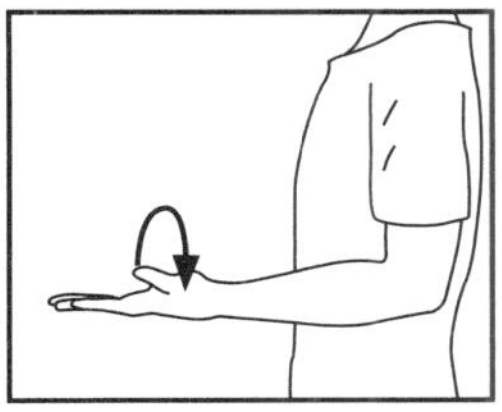

1. ______________________

Name: ______________________________

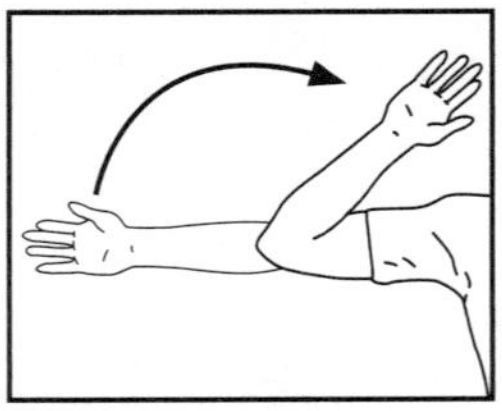

2. ____________________

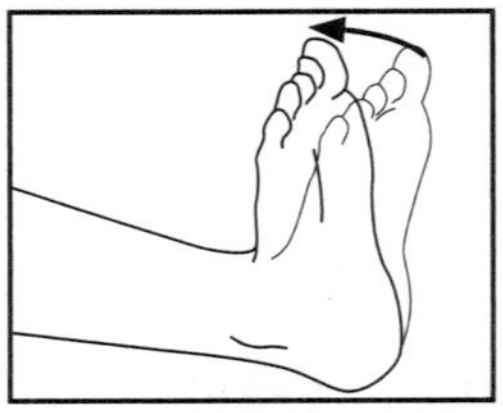

3. ____________________

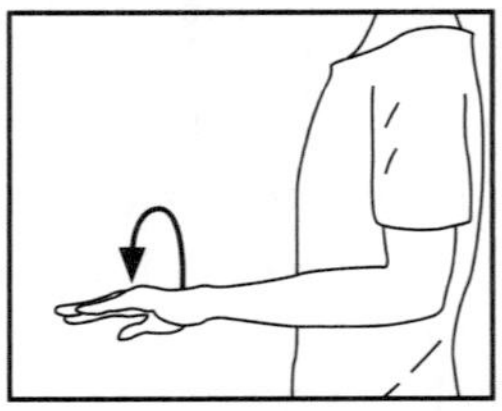

4. ____________________

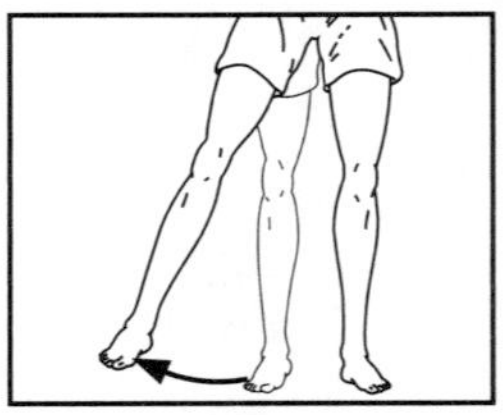

5. ____________________

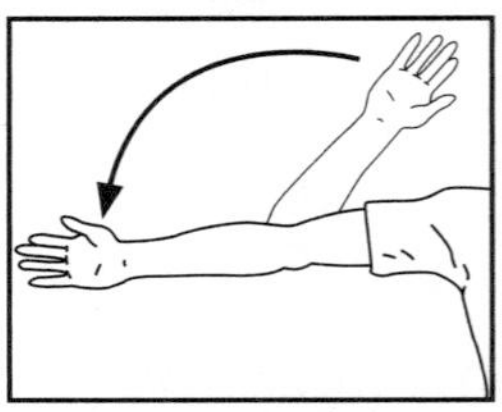

6. ____________________

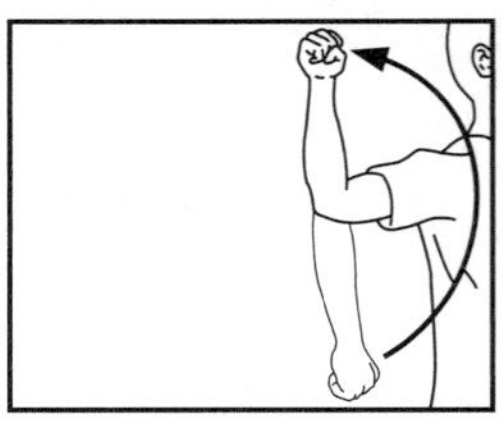

7. ____________________

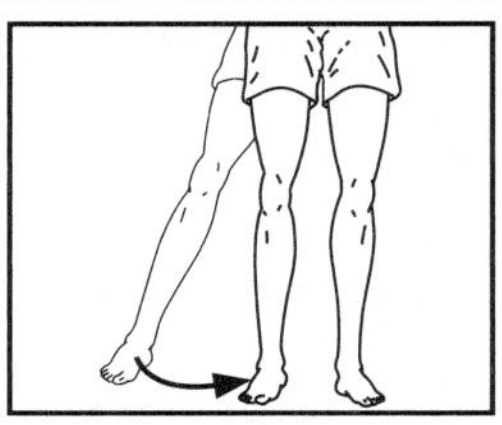

8. ____________________

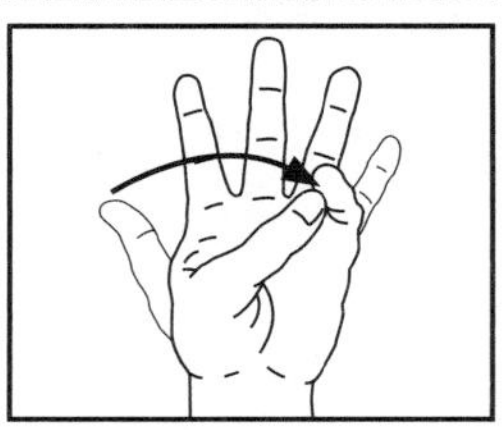

9. ____________________

Multiple Choice

10. In what order should the HHA perform range of motion (ROM) exercises?
    (A) He should start from the feet and work upward.
    (B) He should start from the shoulders and work downward.
    (C) He should start at the hands and work inward.
    (D) He should exercise the arms last.

11. If a client reports pain during ROM exercises, the HHA should
    (A) Continue with the exercises as planned
    (B) Continue, but perform the motion that caused pain more gently
    (C) Stop the exercises and report the pain to his supervisor
    (D) Stop the motion for 1 minute before starting again

12. How many times should each ROM exercise be repeated?
    (A) At least 6 times
    (B) At least 10 times
    (C) At least 12 times
    (D) At least 3 times

5. Explain guidelines for maintaining proper body alignment

Fill in the Blank

1. Observe principles of body ____________________. Remember that proper alignment is based on straight ____________________. ____________________ or rolled or folded ____________________ may be needed to support the small of the back and raise the knees or head in the supine position.

2. Keep body parts in natural ____________________. In a natural hand position, the fingers are slightly ____________________. Use __________ __________ to keep covers from resting on feet for clients in the supine position.

3. Prevent external rotation of _______________. Change _______________ frequently to prevent muscle stiffness and pressure injuries. This should be done at least every _______________ hours.

6. List guidelines for providing basic skin care and preventing pressure injuries

Crossword

Across

2. May be caused by pulling a client across the sheet when transferring him
4. Keeps top sheets from resting on the legs and feet
5. Skin should be kept clean and ________.
6. One type of material that prevents air from circulating, causing the skin to sweat

Down

1. Skin that is _______________ should not be massaged. Massage the healthy skin around it instead.
3. What the bottom sheet on a client's bed must be kept free from
7. At a minimum, the number of hours at which immobile clients should be repositioned

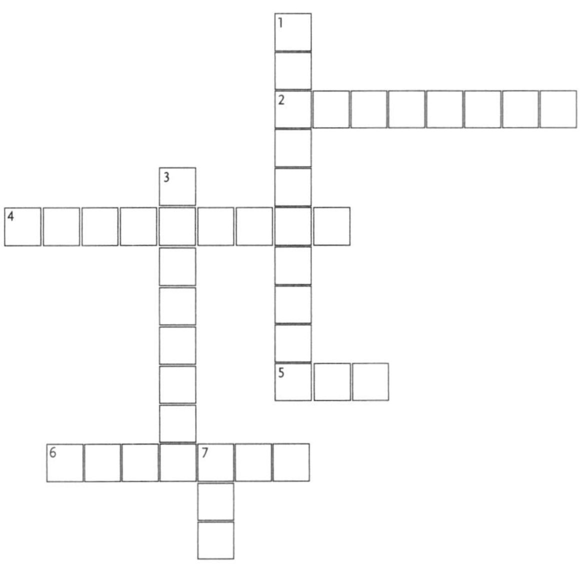

7. Describe guidelines for caring for clients who have fractures or casts

Multiple Choice

1. When caring for a client who has a cast, _______________ the extremity that is in a cast to help stop swelling.
   (A) Lower
   (B) Double bandage
   (C) Elevate
   (D) Shake

2. Keep the cast _______________ at all times.
   (A) Dry
   (B) Wet
   (C) Hot
   (D) Lowered

3. Osteoporosis occurs more frequently in _______________ people.
   (A) Young
   (B) Active
   (C) Elderly
   (D) Diabetic

4. Signs and symptoms of a fracture include
   (A) Moistness at the site
   (B) Cold area at the site
   (C) Swelling at the site
   (D) Dryness at the site

5. Fractures are broken bones and may be caused by
   (A) Excessive fiber
   (B) Asthma
   (C) Osteoporosis
   (D) Too much progesterone

6. Casts that are made of fiberglass are
   (A) Heavy
   (B) Unable to dry properly
   (C) Lightweight
   (D) Less reliable than other types of casts

7. When should a client insert something inside the cast?
   (A) When skin itches
   (B) After the cast dries
   (C) When the cast is wet
   (D) Never

Name: ______________________

8. List guidelines for caring for clients who have had a hip replacement

Complete the Sentence

1. Most fractured hips require *a cast* | *surgery*.
2. The HHA *should* | *should not* perform exercises on the operative leg unless directed otherwise by a supervisor.
3. Preventing *falls* | *ambulation* is an important part of preventing hip fractures.
4. Elderly people heal *quickly* | *slowly*.
5. HHAs *may* | *may not* disconnect a traction assembly if the client requests it.
6. The HHA should begin with the *affected (weaker)* | *unaffected (stronger)* side when dressing a client who is recovering from a hip replacement.
7. With chair or toilet transfers, the *affected (operative)* | *stronger* leg should stand first.

Multiple Choice

8. What does the abbreviation *PWB* stand for?
   (A) Previously weakened bones
   (B) Partial weight-bearing
   (C) Patient's weight before
   (D) Patient wants baths
9. If an HHA sees *NWB* on a client's care plan, the client
   (A) Can support 100 percent of their body weight on a step
   (B) Can support some weight, but not all, on one or both legs
   (C) Is unable to support any weight on one or both legs
   (D) Can use stairs without assistance

9. List ways to adapt the environment for people with physical limitations

Short Answer

Choose an assistive device from Figure 16-27 in the textbook (one you did not choose to answer question 14 in the Chapter Review). Describe how it might help a client who is recovering from or adapting to a physical condition.

____

____

____

____

____

____

____

____

____

____

____

10. Identify reasons clients lose bowel or bladder control

Fill in the Blank

1. When people cannot control the muscles of the bowel or bladder, they are said to have ______________________.
2. A(n) ______________ ______________ placed on the bed helps protect the bed.
3. Clients who are incontinent need to be kept ______________________, ______________________, and free from odor.
4. Urine and feces need to be washed off completely by bathing and proper ______________ care.

5. HHAs should not refer to incontinence briefs or pads as ______________________ because clients are not infants.
6. Clients who are incontinent need ______________________, understanding, and empathy from HHAs.

11. Explain guidelines for assisting with bowel or bladder retraining

Scenarios

Ms. Potter has been recovering from a broken hip. Her recovery is proceeding well, but she has had a problem with urinary incontinence since her injury. Her doctor asked that bladder retraining be added into her care plan. Below are examples of how three HHAs help Ms. Potter with retraining. Read each one and state what the HHA is doing well and/or what he or she should do differently.

1. Hannah, a new HHA, wants to be very professional about the episodes of incontinence. While she is cleaning the bed, she remains very upbeat and friendly and does not mention the incontinence unless Ms. Potter brings it up.

____

____

____

____

____

2. Greta senses Ms. Potter's acute embarrassment, and it makes her nervous. Whenever she has to assist Ms. Potter with retraining efforts, she speaks very little and does not make eye contact with her. She tries to finish her work as quickly as possible to limit Ms. Potter's discomfort.

____

____

____

____

____

3. Pete has been very encouraging and positive with Ms. Potter. He has charted her bathroom schedule. He encourages her to drink more fluids. He makes sure he is nearby to help her during the usual times that she needs to go to the bathroom.

____

____

____

____

____

12. Describe benefits of deep breathing exercises

Short Answer

What can deep breathing exercises help?

____

____

____

____

____

____

____

Name: ______________________________

Please do not
copy our workbook.
Report violations to
legal@hartmanonline.com.

17

Clients with Disabilities

1. Define *disability* and identify common causes of disabilities

Short Answer

1. List three factors that affect how well a person copes with a disability.

____

____

____

____

____

____

____

2. List six diseases and disorders that may cause disability.

____

____

____

____

____

____

____

3. What are two types of disabilities that can be caused by injury to the head or spinal cord?

____

____

____

____

2. Describe daily challenges a person with a disability may face

Short Answer

List five daily challenges a person with a disability may face.

____

____

____

____

____

____

____

3. Define terms related to disabilities and explain why they are important

Short Answer

1. How does using person-first language relate to providing person-centered care?

____

____

____

____

____

____

____

Name: ______________________

2. To avoid using terms that are offensive to a client with a disability, what should the HHA do?

____

____

____

____

____

____

4. Identify social and emotional needs of persons with disabilities

Fill in the Blank

1. Basic psychosocial needs include independence, social interaction, acceptance, a sense of worth, and ______________________.
2. HHAs should treat all clients with ______________________.
3. HHAs should not push clients beyond their ______________________.
4. HHAs can give clients ______________________ to show what they can do by themselves.

5. Explain how a disability may affect sexuality and intimacy

True or False

1. ____ Most people who have a disability do not experience sexual desires.
2. ____ For a person with a disability, the ability to meet sexual needs may be limited.
3. ____ People in wheelchairs are unable to have sexual relationships.
4. ____ It is important for an HHA not to judge any sexual behavior they see.

6. Identify skills that can be applied to clients with disabilities

Short Answer

List three skills that can be applied to working with clients with disabilities.

____

____

____

____

7. List five goals to work toward when assisting clients who have disabilities

Fill in the Blank

1. Promote self-care and ______________________.
2. Ensure the client's ______________________.
3. Promote the client's health and ______________________.
4. Maintain the client's ______________________ and self-worth.
5. Maintain the ______________________ of the client's household.

8. Identify five qualities of excellent service needed by clients with disabilities

Short Answer

List the five qualities of excellent service needed by clients with disabilities.

____

____

____

____

____

____

____

9. Explain how to adapt personal care procedures to meet the needs of clients with disabilities

True or False

1. ____ Children who have Down syndrome do not appear physically different from any other child.
2. ____ Developmental disabilities normally appear and are diagnosed when a person is middle-aged.
3. ____ The most common type of developmental disorder is intellectual disability.
4. ____ Having an intellectual disability is the same as having a mental health disorder.
5. ____ Clients who have an intellectual disability have the same emotional and physical needs that others have.
6. ____ Speech impairment is one possible effect of cerebral palsy.
7. ____ It is possible that some babies born with spina bifida will be able to walk and will experience no lasting disabilities.
8. ____ One sign of autism spectrum disorder is that the child does not engage in pretend play.
9. ____ Intensely focused interests can be a sign of autism spectrum disorder.
10. ____ Treatment for autism spectrum disorder should be started early and tailored to the individual.

10. List important changes to report and document for a client with disabilities

Short Answer

1. What should the HHA do if he notices that a client is unable to perform a task that she was previously able to do?

____

____

____

____

2. Give two signs of depression that should be reported.

____

____

____

____

Name: ______________________

Please do not
copy our workbook.
Report violations to
legal@hartmanonline.com.

18

Mental Health and Mental Health Disorders

1. Identify seven characteristics of mental health

Short Answer

1. Define *mental health.*

____
____
____
____
____
____

2. List seven characteristics of a person who is mentally healthy.

____
____
____
____
____
____
____
____
____

2. Discuss causes of mental health disorders

Complete the Sentence

1. Mental health disorders *may* | *do not ever* have physical causes.
2. A mental health disorder *does not affect* | *disrupts* a person's ability to function in the family, home, or community.
3. A personal crisis, temporary physical changes in the brain, side effects from medications, interactions among medications, certain acute medical conditions, or a severe change in the environment may cause *permanent* | *temporary* signs and symptoms that mimic a mental health disorder.
4. Substance use disorder *is unrelated to* | *can cause* mental health disorders.

3. Distinguish between fact and fallacy concerning mental health disorders

True or False

1. ____ A fallacy is a false belief.
2. ____ People who have a mental health disorder have the power to be well if they really want to.
3. ____ People who have a mental health disorder may not be able to control their emotions and responses.
4. ____ An intellectual disability is a type of mental health disorder.

Name: ______________________

Mental Health and Mental Health Disorders

4. Explain the connection between mental and physical wellness

Short Answer

Briefly describe why mental health is important to physical health.

5. List guidelines for communicating with clients who have a mental health disorder

Short Answer

1. When communicating with a client who has a mental health disorder, why is it important for the HHA to treat the client as an individual and to tailor the HHA's style of communication to the situation?

2. Why do you think it is important for the HHA not to talk to adults as if they were children?

6. Identify and define common defense mechanisms

Short Answer

Read each description below and identify the defense mechanism that is being used.

1. When Aaron's mother yells at him for breaking a vase in the living room, he goes into his room and yells at his stuffed bear.

2. When Gia was 10, she was very badly injured in a car accident. She was in the hospital for almost 3 months, but now she tries not to think about that time.

3. When Marco accuses his little sister Ana of having a crush on the boy who sits next to her in class, she blushes and cries, "I do not!"

4. When Esther was 42, her husband died of lung cancer. After his death, she got out the quilt she used to sleep with as a child and curled up in bed with it for days.

5. Wayne is fixing a leaky sink in the bathroom. When his wife teases him about taking a long time to fix it, he replies, "It's not my fault. I can't concentrate on anything with you bothering me all the time."

7. Describe types of mental health disorders

Multiple Choice

1. Uneasiness, worry, or fear, often about a situation or condition, is called
   (A) Anxiety
   (B) Withdrawal
   (C) Fatigue
   (D) Apathy

2. An intense, irrational fear of or anxiety about an object, place, or situation is called a
   (A) Depressive episode
   (B) Delusion
   (C) Phobia
   (D) Hallucination

3. Which type of mental health disorder is most commonly associated with suicide in older adults?
   (A) Anxiety
   (B) Apathy
   (C) Irritability
   (D) Depression

4. Which of the following means a lack of interest in activities?
   (A) Guilt
   (B) Depression
   (C) Apathy
   (D) Delusion

5. A persistent false belief, such as a person believing that someone else is controlling his thoughts, is a
   (A) Defense mechanism
   (B) Delusion
   (C) Phobia
   (D) Hallucination

6. A disorder that is characterized by recurring intrusive behavior or thoughts, such as repeatedly checking that the door is locked, is
   (A) Major depressive disorder
   (B) Panic disorder
   (C) Obsessive-compulsive disorder
   (D) Manic disorder

7. Experiencing periods of extreme activity or excitement along with periods of deep depression or sadness is characterized as
   (A) Major depressive disorder
   (B) Panic disorder
   (C) Posttraumatic stress disorder
   (D) Bipolar disorder

8. What may cause posttraumatic stress disorder?
   (A) Smoking and using illegal substances
   (B) Exercising infrequently
   (C) Eating a diet high in sugar and processed foods
   (D) Experiencing violence or poverty

8. Explain common treatments for mental health disorders

True or False

1. ____ Mental health disorders cannot be treated.

2. ____ Medication and psychotherapy are commonly used to treat mental health disorders.

3. ____ HHAs are usually responsible for prescribing medication for clients who have a mental health disorder.

4. ____ Medication can allow those who have a mental health disorder to function more completely.

5. ____ A common type of psychotherapy used to treat anxiety disorders is electroconvulsive (electroshock) therapy.

6. ____ For a person who has trouble regulating their emotions, dialectical behavior therapy may be used.

9. Explain the home health aide's role in caring for clients who have a mental health disorder

Short Answer

List four care guidelines for clients who have a mental health disorder.

____

____

____

____

____

____

____

____

____

____

10. Identify important observations that should be made and reported

True or False

1. ____ It is important for the HHA to report to the supervisor if a client who has a mental health disorder stops taking her medication.

2. ____ As long as a client is joking when talking about suicide, the HHA does not need to report it.

11. List the signs of substance use disorder

Multiple Choice

1. Circle any of the following substances that can be abused:
   (A) Alcohol
   (B) Cigarettes
   (C) Illegal drugs
   (D) Glue
   (E) Paint
   (F) Prescription medicine

2. A client has been acting a little strangely lately. She gets upset very easily, and her eyes are always red. She does not eat much, and sometimes her HHA can smell alcohol on her breath, even in the morning. What is the best response by the HHA?
   (A) Confront the client about what the HHA has noticed.
   (B) Contact Alcoholics Anonymous to get advice on how to handle the situation.
   (C) Document the HHA's observations and report them to her supervisor.
   (D) Search the client's cabinets for alcohol and throw away any alcohol found.

3. Which of the following statements about opioid medication is true?
   (A) All opioids are legally prescribed by providers.
   (B) When a person takes opioids, her tolerance for the drug decreases, requiring lower doses of the medication.
   (C) Opioids are powerful pain medications that pose a high risk for addiction.
   (D) Opioids are available over the counter, without a prescription.

19

New Mothers, Infants, and Children

1. Explain the growth of home care for new mothers and infants

True or False

1. ____ Most new mothers stay in the hospital for several days to a week after childbirth.
2. ____ Bed rest is ordered if a woman shows signs of early labor.
3. ____ HHAs may be needed when an expectant mother is put on bed rest by her doctor.
4. ____ New mothers today are generally more energetic when they come home than women in the past.
5. ____ Bed rest may help prevent labor from starting before the baby is ready to be born.
6. ____ Natural childbirth techniques have been a factor in how long new mothers stay in the hospital after delivery.

2. Identify common neonatal disorders

Short Answer

List three common neonatal disorders.

____

____

____

____

____

____

3. Explain how to provide postpartum care

Fill in the Blank

Use this list of words and phrases to fill in the blanks in the following sentences. Use each word or phrase only once.

bathing	Cesarean section
diapering	episiotomy
feeding	housekeeping
lactation	lochia
monitor	pink
red	

1. An incision sometimes made in the perineum during vaginal delivery to enlarge the vaginal opening for the baby's head is a(n) ______________________________.
2. The HHA may need to monitor the amount and color of the new mother's ______________________________, which is the vaginal flow that occurs after giving birth.
3. Basic care for the baby includes ______________________________, ______________________________, and ______________________________.
4. The HHA may be required to do light ______________________________ to help the new mother.
5. A surgical procedure in which the baby is delivered through an incision in the mother's abdomen is called a(n) ______________________________.

Name: ____________________

6. HHAs may be asked to ______________________ the equipment if the baby is receiving oxygen.
7. During the first several days after childbirth, the color of lochia usually changes from bright __________ to __________.
8. If a new mother needs help with breastfeeding, a(n) ______________________ consultant can help.

4. List important observations to report and document

Short Answer

Read this scenario and answer the questions that follow.

The HHA arrives at a client's house at 8 a.m. to care for baby Eric, a 2-day-old newborn, and finds the house cluttered, the new mother Anne in a sitz bath, and baby Eric in the crib crying. The mother is also crying and says she got "no sleep last night." What course of action should the HHA take? How would the HHA document this?

____

____

____

____

____

____

____

____

____

____

____

____

____

____

____

5. Explain guidelines for safely handling a baby

Labeling

Label the type of hold shown in each figure.

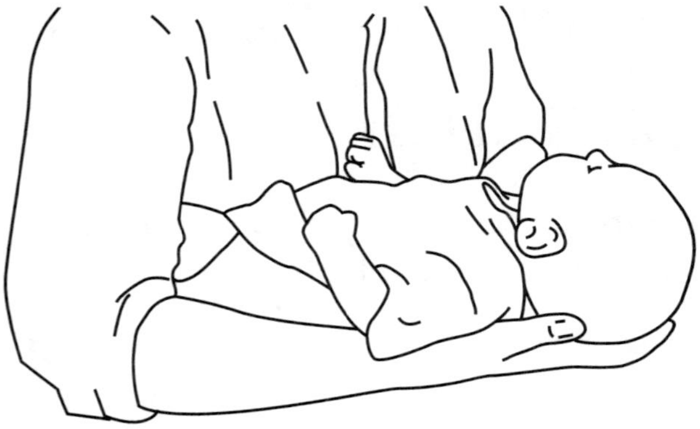

1. ______________________________

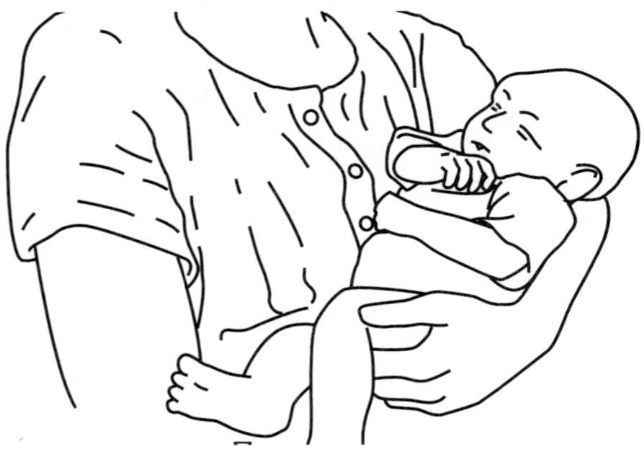

2. ______________________________

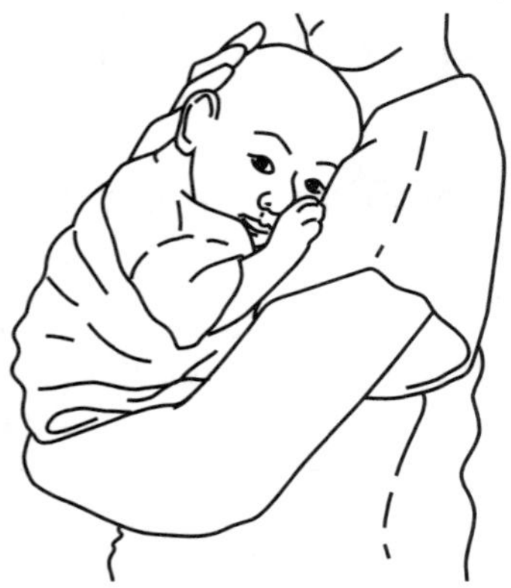

3. ______________________________

6. Describe guidelines for assisting with feeding a baby

Multiple Choice

1. If the baby does not latch on to the nipple right away, the mother should stroke his
   (A) Toes
   (B) Elbow
   (C) Cheek
   (D) Forehead

2. Many professionals recommend that mothers try breastfeeding for ________ week(s) before deciding whether to continue or stop.
   (A) 5
   (B) 10
   (C) 1
   (D) 2

3. Powdered formula is sold in
   (A) Crates
   (B) Cans
   (C) Sterilized pitchers
   (D) Squeezable pouches

4. The cheapest formula is usually
   (A) Ready-to-use
   (B) Concentrated liquid
   (C) Powdered
   (D) Ready-made

5. A good position for breastfeeding is
   (A) Lying face down on the bed
   (B) Sitting upright in a comfortable chair
   (C) Rocking rapidly in a chair
   (D) Bending over the crib

6. Before feeding, the HHA should check the temperature of the formula on her wrist. It should feel
   (A) Warm
   (B) Hot
   (C) Cold
   (D) Boiling

7. The mother can break the suction of a nursing baby by
   (A) Pulling down the baby's ears
   (B) Putting her finger in the baby's mouth
   (C) Sucking on the baby's toes
   (D) Tickling the baby

8. Which of the following is best for bottle-fed newborns?
   (A) Whole milk
   (B) Infant formula
   (C) Fruit smoothies
   (D) Skim milk

7. Explain guidelines for bathing and changing a baby

True or False

1. ____ The HHA should wear disposable gloves when changing or bathing a baby.
2. ____ Leaving a diaper off for a few minutes when changing the baby can help prevent diaper rash.
3. ____ The proper way to test a baby's bath temperature is by dipping the baby's hand in it.
4. ____ Moisture contributes to diaper rash.
5. ____ It is okay for the HHA to take both hands off the baby if it is for less than a minute.
6. ____ Children generally wear diapers until they are 8 to 12 months old.
7. ____ Newborns will need between 8 and 12 diaper changes in 24 hours.
8. ____ The HHA should apply baby powder to the baby's body after giving the baby a bath.
9. ____ It is a sign of a medical problem if a newborn baby has a loose bowel movement with every feeding.
10. ____ Babies should be changed frequently to avoid diaper rash.

8. Identify how to measure weight and length of a baby

Multiple Choice

1. When weighing a baby, the HHA should
   (A) Keep one hand on the baby at all times
   (B) Step back from the scale after the baby is on it so as not to interfere with an accurate measurement
   (C) Place the scale on the floor to see if the baby will crawl onto it
   (D) Stand the baby up on the scale for an accurate weight

2. How can a baby's length be determined?
   (A) By standing the baby up against a wall, making a pencil mark at the top of his head, and measuring the height of the mark
   (B) By holding the baby against the HHA's leg and measuring how high the baby's head reaches
   (C) By placing the baby on paper, making pencil marks at the head and heel, and measuring the distance between the marks
   (D) By putting the baby on a standing scale and lowering the measuring rod until it rests flat on the baby's head

9. Explain guidelines for special care

Matching

1. ____ Apnea
2. ____ Circumcision
3. _____ Feeding pump
4. ____ Oxygen
5. ____ Umbilical cord

(A) The cord that connects the baby to the placenta

(B) The surgical removal of part of the foreskin of the penis

(C) The state of not breathing

(D) Given to some babies who have breathing problems; considered a medication

(E) Method of giving some preterm and low-birth-weight babies nutrition through a tube

10. Identify special needs of children and describe how children respond to stress

Short Answer

1. List some examples of physiological needs that children have.

____
____
____
____
____
____

2. List an example of a mental need that children have.

____
____
____

3. List four examples of emotional needs that children have.

____
____
____
____
____
____
____

4. List five reasons that children may experience stress.

____
____
____

____

____

____

____

5. List five factors that influence the way in which children respond to stress.

____

____

____

____

____

____

____

____

6. In what ways might school-age children react to stress?

____

____

____

____

____

____

____

7. In what negative ways might adolescents react to stress?

____

____

____

____

____

____

____

11. List symptoms of common childhood illnesses and the required care

Fill in the Blank

1. ______________________________, cleaning, and disinfection are the best ways to prevent infection.
2. Frequent loose or watery bowel movements are called ______________________.
3. Children with diarrhea may experience ______________________, thus doctors may recommend electrolyte-replacement drinks.
4. In general, children should not be given ______________________, because it has been associated with serious disorders.
5. Treatment for a fever includes acetaminophen or ibuprofen or a lukewarm bath or ______________________.
6. Doctors usually recommend that children resume their normal, well-balanced diet within __________ hours of having diarrhea.
7. Rest and ______________________ are recommended for fevers.
8. Too much acetaminophen can cause ______________________ damage.

12. Identify guidelines for working with children

Scenarios

Read the following scenarios and decide how to respond.

1. Zack and his older brother Lee have just returned home from school. Zack is upset because he did not win a prize for his science project, but his brother did. He cried at school, and some of the other kids made fun of him. He becomes visibly distressed again as he relates this story to the HHA at his home. What would be the best response by the HHA?

____

____

Name: ______________________

____

2. The HHA notices that Doug has been withdrawn all afternoon. He did not go outside to play after school, and at dinner, he refuses to eat anything. He makes comments such as "Nobody cares about me." What would be the best response by the HHA?

____

13. List the signs of child abuse and neglect and know how to report them

Short Answer

1. Psychological abuse of children includes

____

2. Sexual abuse of children includes

____

3. Child neglect is

____

20

Dying, Death, and Hospice

1. Discuss the stages of grief

Multiple Choice

Read each scenario below and choose which stage of grief the person described is experiencing.

1. Mr. Cane was told 2 years ago that a tumor in his brain was inoperable and would eventually be fatal. Since that time, he has visited many specialists. Despite receiving the same diagnosis from every doctor, he continues to seek further opinions, insisting that each doctor try to remove the tumor. Which stage of grief is Mr. Cane in?
   (A) Denial
   (B) Anger
   (C) Bargaining
   (D) Depression
   (E) Acceptance

2. Mrs. Tyler is dying of heart disease. One day as her HHA, Makayla, is assisting her with personal care, Mrs. Tyler lashes out at her. She tells Makayla that she is a dumb girl who is wasting her life and does not deserve the many years she has left to live. Which stage of grief is Mrs. Tyler in?
   (A) Denial
   (B) Anger
   (C) Bargaining
   (D) Depression
   (E) Acceptance

3. Mr. Lopez is dying of AIDS. He has called his friends to say goodbye and has discussed with his family the kind of memorial service he would like them to arrange. Which stage of grief is Mr. Lopez in?
   (A) Denial
   (B) Anger
   (C) Bargaining
   (D) Depression
   (E) Acceptance

4. Ms. Corke has always been lively and happy. Since she learned that she has Lou Gehrig disease, however, her mood has changed drastically. Although she is still healthy enough to do activities, she rarely leaves her bedroom or even changes out of her pajamas. Which stage of grief is Ms. Corke in?
   (A) Denial
   (B) Anger
   (C) Bargaining
   (D) Depression
   (E) Acceptance

5. Mr. Celasco has had lung cancer for several years. During that time, he has tried to quit smoking but has been unsuccessful. When he finds out that there are no further treatments for him to try, he pledges that he will give up smoking in exchange for a few more years of life. Which stage of grief is Mr. Celasco in?
   (A) Denial
   (B) Anger
   (C) Bargaining
   (D) Depression
   (E) Acceptance

Name: ____________________

2. Describe the grief process

Multiple Choice

Read each scenario below and choose which reaction to a loved one's death each person is experiencing.

1. Malcolm's wife died during the birth of their second daughter. Malcolm is so upset with her for abandoning him and the children that he cannot even stand to hear her name spoken. Which reaction is Malcolm experiencing?
   (A) Loneliness
   (B) Denial
   (C) Anger
   (D) Guilt
   (E) Sadness

2. Shanice's mother had been ill for many years before she died when Shanice was 15 years old. After her death, Shanice remembers how she used to resent helping her mother around the house and wishes that she had been kinder and more cheerful. Which reaction is she having?
   (A) Anger
   (B) Sadness
   (C) Guilt
   (D) Denial
   (E) Relief

3. Melinda's grandmother, to whom she was very close, died after a long illness on Sunday afternoon. On Monday morning, Melinda's mother is astonished to find Melinda cheerfully getting ready for school as she does every Monday morning. Which reaction is Melinda having?
   (A) Loneliness
   (B) Denial
   (C) Relief
   (D) Guilt
   (E) Regret

4. Micah's best friend, Lawrence, died of cancer at the age of 45. Whenever Micah spends time with the friends that they had in common, he is reminded of Lawrence and feels sad. He is not as close to his other friends as he was to Lawrence, and he feels he has no one to confide in since Lawrence is gone. Which reaction is he having?
   (A) Shock
   (B) Denial
   (C) Anger
   (D) Loneliness
   (E) Guilt

5. Theresa's 9-year-old son went to a pool party for a friend's birthday and accidentally drowned. Theresa has been unable to forgive herself for letting him go to the party. Which reaction is she having?
   (A) Anger
   (B) Loneliness
   (C) Denial
   (D) Guilt
   (E) Shock

6. Casey's brother was killed suddenly in a car accident. He is surprised that he seems to feel very little emotion regarding the death. Which reaction is Casey having?
   (A) Relief
   (B) Shock
   (C) Guilt
   (D) Anger
   (E) Regret

7. When Elizabeth's boyfriend was killed by a drunk driver on his way home one night, Elizabeth was inconsolable. She has stopped seeing her friends and stays in her room crying for hours at a time. Which reaction is she having?
   (A) Anger
   (B) Sadness
   (C) Guilt
   (D) Denial
   (E) Regret

8. Marcela's father recently died after battling heart failure for many years. When he got sicker, Marcela had to take a leave of absence from work to help deal with his care, which greatly affected her income and caused her worry. She found herself resenting him at times. After he died, Marcela felt sad, but she also thinks about how she is free to make her own decisions about her life again. Which reaction is she having?
   (A) Anger
   (B) Denial
   (C) Relief
   (D) Guilt
   (E) Loneliness

3. Discuss how feelings and attitudes about death differ

Short Answer

1. Have you ever experienced the death of a loved one? If so, what are some of the emotions you felt?

____

____

____

____

____

____

____

____

2. What, if any, religious beliefs do you subscribe to? How do they influence your feelings about death? If you do not have any religious or spiritual beliefs, what are your feelings about death?

____

____

____

____

____

____

____

____

3. What cultural background do you have? What cultures are you familiar with? Briefly describe how your culture or other cultures you are familiar with feel about death.

____

____

____

____

____

____

____

____

____

4. Discuss how to care for a client who is dying

True or False

1. ____ Advance directives do not need to be honored if the medical professional feels he can save the person's life.
2. ____ Listening to a client who is dying is an important thing that an HHA can do.
3. ____ Hearing is usually the last sense to leave the body, so the HHA should continue to speak in a normal tone.
4. ____ When a person is dying, he no longer needs skin care.
5. ____ Keeping the room lighting low is best for a client who is dying.
6. ____ It is important for HHAs to observe clients for signs of pain, as they may not be able to communicate that they are in pain.

Name: ______________________

7. ____ Back massage is one way to help clients who are in pain.
8. ____ It is best to keep a client who is dying isolated (by himself).
9. ____ To help a client who is dying to think positively, the HHA can tell the client that he could still recover.

5. Explain legal rights for clients who are dying and describe ways to promote dignity

Short Answer

1. List three legal rights that must be honored when working with clients who are dying.

____

____

____

2. Look at *The Dying Person's Bill of Rights* on page 356 of your textbook. Pick three rights that you feel would be most important to you. Briefly describe why they would be important to you.

____

____

____

____

____

____

____

____

____

____

____

____

____

____

6. Define the goals of a hospice program and identify guidelines for hospice work

Multiple Choice

1. Hospice care is the term for compassionate care given to
   (A) Clients who have respiratory diseases
   (B) Clients who are dying
   (C) Clients with Parkinson disease
   (D) Clients with developmental disabilities
2. Hospice care encourages clients to
   (A) Allow hospice care teams to handle all care decisions
   (B) Allow lawyers to make care decisions
   (C) Allow doctors to make care decisions
   (D) Participate in their own care as much as possible
3. Hospice goals focus on
   (A) Recovery of the dying person
   (B) Comfort and dignity of the dying person
   (C) Curing the dying person's disease
   (D) Creating a will and other legal documents for the dying person
4. Focusing on pain relief, controlling symptoms, and preventing complications is called ________ care.
   (A) Palliative
   (B) Personal
   (C) Professional
   (D) Pediatric

Short Answer

5. List seven guidelines that are helpful for hospice work.

____

____

____

____

____

____

____

____

____

6. How do you alleviate stress in your life?

____

____

____

____

____

____

____

____

____

____

7. What are three ways you can take care of yourself?

____

____

____

____

____

____

____

____

____

____

____

7. Explain common signs of approaching death

Short Answer

Place a check mark (✓) beside the signs of approaching death.

1. ____ High blood pressure
2. ____ Fever
3. ____ Cold, pale skin
4. ____ Disorientation
5. ____ Healthy skin tone
6. ____ Heightened sense of touch
7. ____ Impaired speech
8. ____ Incontinence
9. ____ Perspiration
10. ____ Strong pulse

8. Describe postmortem care

Multiple Choice

1. After death, the muscles in the body become
   (A) Warm and relaxed
   (B) Bendable
   (C) Stiff and rigid
   (D) Hot and tense

2. Caring for a body after death is called
   (A) Postmortem care
   (B) Mortician care
   (C) Funeral home care
   (D) Before-burial care

3. After death, the HHA should place drainage pads under the body. These pads are most often needed
   (A) Under the arms
   (B) Under the head and/or the perineum
   (C) Under the axillary area
   (D) Under the feet

4. If family members would like to remain with their loved one's body after death, the HHA should
   (A) Let them do so
   (B) Inform them that the HHA needs to ask the doctor first
   (C) Ask them to perform the postmortem care since they are staying with the body
   (D) Talk to them about the importance of organ donation

Name: ______________________________

9. Understand and respect different postmortem practices

Complete the Sentence

1. People grieve *in many different ways* | *mostly in the same way.*
2. Religious beliefs *may* | *do not* influence what family members do after a client has died.
3. The overall mood at a wake is *not necessarily* | *most often* sad or somber.
4. Having a(n) *open* | *closed* casket means the preserved body will be displayed to others.
5. Some people will choose to be *embalmed* | *cremated*, which means the body is burned until it is reduced to ashes.
6. Readings of *scripture and prayers* | *philosophical excerpts* are more likely at the funeral of a client who was an atheist.
7. The use of a shroud or biodegradable casket is associated with a *natural burial* | *viewing.*
8. An HHA should *remain respectful of* | *try to guide* rituals that take place after a client has died.

21
Clean, Safe, and Healthy Environments

1. Describe how housekeeping affects physical and psychological well-being

Short Answer

What are some reasons that HHAs should maintain orderly, clean households for their clients?

____

____

____

____

____

____

____

____

____

____

2. List qualities needed to manage a home and describe general housekeeping guidelines

True or False

1. ____ The HHA's primary responsibility is to clean the client's kitchen.
2. ____ The HHA should expect that all members of the household will be able to help with housekeeping.
3. ____ The HHA will need to be flexible with regard to household maintenance.
4. ____ Vacuuming is not part of an HHA's duties.
5. ____ Using proper body mechanics when performing housekeeping activities helps prevent injury.
6. ____ It is important for HHAs to be sensitive to each client's customs and beliefs.
7. ____ The HHA will need to use cleaning materials and methods that are approved by clients and their families.
8. ____ The HHA should clean up and straighten up after every activity.
9. ____ One HHA responsibility is observing for infestation of insects and animals.

3. Describe cleaning products and equipment

Complete the Sentence

1. *Abrasive* | *All-purpose* cleaners can be used for many purposes and on several types of surfaces.
2. Bleach should never be combined with *ammonia* | *water*.
3. A *dust cloth* | *sponge* is usually used to soften and remove soil on washable surfaces.
4. Vacuum cleaner bags should be checked *annually* | *often*.
5. Cleaning products *are guaranteed never to cause harm* | *can be dangerous if used incorrectly*.

Name: ______________________________

6. Common household items that may be used to create environmentally safe, nontoxic cleaning solutions include *bleach and ammonia* | *white vinegar and lemon juice.*

7. Baking soda can be used as a *scouring powder* | *disinfectant.*

4. Describe proper cleaning methods for living areas, kitchens, bathrooms, and storage areas

Multiple Choice

1. Examples of essential items that should be kept close by the client include
   (A) Eyeglasses
   (B) Potato chips
   (C) Nail polish
   (D) Cosmetics

2. Falls and accidents in the home are frequently caused by
   (A) Contaminated counters
   (B) Wet floors
   (D) Full trash containers
   (D) Leftover food scraps

3. In the kitchen, diseases may be transmitted by
   (A) Soap
   (B) Medications
   (C) Contaminated food surfaces
   (D) Bleach

4. Unless the client has allergies, it is a good idea for the HHA to dust this frequently:
   (A) Five times a week
   (B) Once a week
   (C) Once every 2 months
   (D) Twice a month

5. In order to remove odors, the HHA can use
   (A) Flour
   (B) Baking soda
   (C) Sugar
   (D) Baking powder

6. Dishes may be sterilized by
   (A) Using a dishwasher
   (B) Using cold water
   (C) Using an oven cleaner
   (D) Drying them with a dish towel

7. How often should the HHA dispose of garbage?
   (A) Daily
   (B) Weekly
   (C) Monthly
   (D) Every 2 weeks

8. Basic bathroom hygiene includes
   (A) Washing from dirty areas to clean areas
   (B) Placing soiled towels on the bathroom sink
   (C) Cleaning the tub and shower after each use
   (D) Leaving toothbrushes in the sink

9. Instead of glass cleaner, the HHA can mix water and _____ to clean glass.
   (A) Wine
   (B) Vinegar
   (C) Apple juice
   (D) Spray starch

10. In what environments do mold and mildew grow best?
    (A) In cold areas
    (B) In dry places
    (C) In warm, moist places
    (D) In windy areas

11. Living area floors and rugs should be vacuumed at least
    (A) Once a month
    (B) Twice a week
    (C) Once a week
    (D) Once a day

12. Which of the following materials is commonly recycled?
    (A) Wood
    (B) Plastic
    (C) Polyester
    (D) Marble

13. A nontoxic solution that can be used to remove grease on surfaces is:
    (A) Acetone solution
    (B) Ammonia solution
    (C) Bleach solution
    (D) Lemon juice solution

5. Describe how to prepare a cleaning schedule

Short Answer

Create a sample cleaning schedule for a client who is immobile.

Immediately:

____

____

____

____

____

Daily:

____

____

____

____

____

Weekly:

____

____

____

____

____

Monthly:

____

____

____

____

____

Less often:

____

____

____

____

____

____

6. List special housekeeping procedures to use when infection is present

Fill in the Blank

1. ______________________ any surfaces that come into contact with body fluids, such as ______________________, urinals, and toilets.
2. Frequently remove ______________________ containing used tissues.
3. Keep any ______________________ of urine, stool, or sputum in double bags away from food.
4. ______________________ dishes and utensils should be used for the client.
5. Wash dishes in hot, soapy water with ______________________, and rinse in ______________________ water.
6. ______________________ the client's bathroom daily.

Name: ____________________

7. Explain how to do laundry and care for clothes

Crossword

Across

3. Washing cycle used for sturdy permanent press items and cottons
4. Chemical that whitens clothing and removes stains
5. Substance used to dilute bleach
6. Delicate fabric requires ____________________ time in the dryer.
7. Washing cycle used for delicate items
8. One way to reduce these is to fold clothes immediately after they are dried
9. Water temperature used for whites and towels

Down

1. Type of bleach used on washable fabrics; most effective in hot water
2. Parts of a shirt that are ironed first, after collars, cuffs, and garment facings
5. The safest water temperature for most garments
6. Cleaned every time the dryer is used

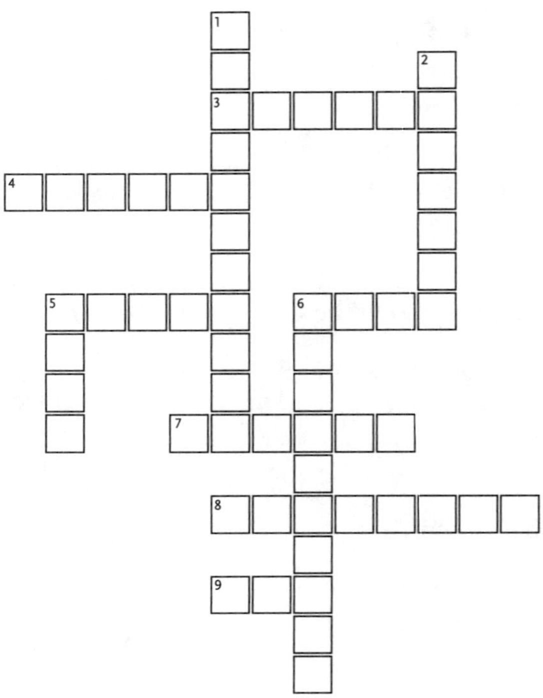

8. List special laundry precautions to use when infection is present

True or False

1. ____ It is best to use cold water when doing laundry for a client who has an infectious disease.
2. ____ The HHA should wear gloves when doing the laundry for a client who has an infectious disease.
3. ____ Dirty laundry should be shaken to remove dirt before putting it in the washing machine.
4. ____ The HHA should keep the client's laundry separate from other family members' laundry.
5. ____ Dirty laundry should remain in the client's room as long as possible so as to avoid contamination of the rest of the house.
6. ____ Agency-approved disinfectants should be used in loads of laundry.

9. List guidelines for teaching housekeeping skills to clients' family members

Short Answer

Read the following scenario and decide how to respond.

Dave, an HHA, is explaining to Mrs. Crawford's family how to protect against infectious diseases when doing the laundry and cleaning the kitchen. He has written a long list of instructions, and when he is done explaining, two family members still seem confused about some key points. How should Dave respond in this situation?

____

____

____

____

____

____

10. Discuss the importance of sleep and explain why careful bedmaking is important

Multiple Choice

1. Why is it important for HHAs to change bed linens often?
   (A) To get clients out of their beds and moving around
   (B) To rotate clean sheets evenly
   (C) To keep skills up-to-date
   (D) To prevent infection and to promote comfort

2. When removing dirty linen, the HHA should
   (A) Fold it so that the soiled area is outside
   (B) Roll it so that the soiled area is inside
   (C) Gather it in a bunch
   (D) Shake it to remove particles

3. A bed made with the bedspread and blankets in place is called a(n)
   (A) Open bed
   (B) Stretcher bed
   (C) Closed bed
   (D) Completed bed

11. Identify hazardous household materials

Short Answer

Identify five hazardous household materials.

Name: ______________________________

Please do not
copy our workbook.
Report violations to
legal@hartmanonline.com.

22

Clients' Nutritional Needs

1. Describe the importance of proper nutrition and list the six basic nutrients

Short Answer

Write the letter of the correct nutrient beside each description. Use a W for water, C for carbohydrates, P for protein, F for fats, V for vitamins, and M for minerals. Letters may be used more than once.

1. ____ Sources include vegetarian and vegan meat substitutes.
2. ____ A person can survive only a few days without this.
3. ____ These build bones and help in blood formation.
4. ____ These add flavor to food and help to absorb certain vitamins.
5. ____ Examples include bread, cereal, and potatoes.
6. ____ They are essential for tissue growth and repair.
7. ____ The body cannot make most of these nutrients; they must be obtained by eating certain foods.
8. ____ They provide fiber, which is necessary for bowel elimination.
9. ____ They may come from plant sources such as olives and nuts.
10. ____ This is the most essential nutrient for life.
11. ____ Categories include monounsaturated and saturated.
12. ____ This helps to maintain body temperature through perspiration.
13. ____ These can be fat-soluble or water-soluble.
14. ____ These help the body store energy.
15. ____ Iron and magnesium are examples.

2. Describe the USDA's MyPlate

Short Answer

The USDA developed the MyPlate icon and website to help promote healthy eating practices. Looking at the MyPlate icon below, fill in the food groups.

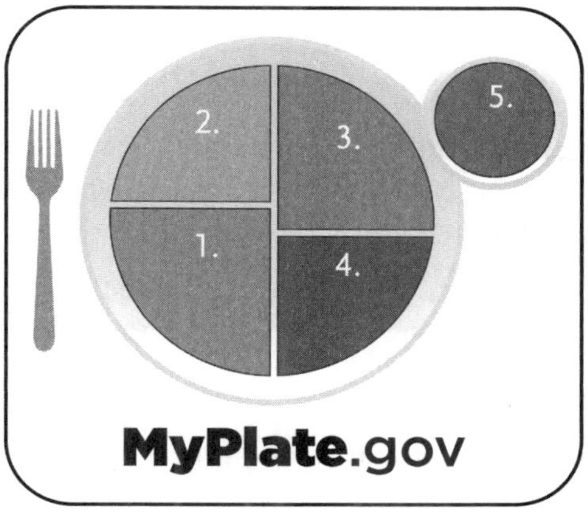

1. ______________________
2. ______________________
3. ______________________
4. ______________________
5. ______________________

Short Answer

Read the following descriptions and mark which each is describing—V for vegetables, F for fruits, G for grains, P for protein, and D for dairy. Letters will be used more than once.

6. ____ This group includes foods that retain their calcium content, such as yogurt and cheese.

Name: ______________________

7. ____ Wheat, rice, oats, cornmeal, and barley are examples.

8. ____ Plant sources of this include beans and soy products.

9. ____ Eating seafood twice a week in place of meat or poultry is recommended for this group.

10. ____ Most choices from this group should be fat-free or low-fat.

11. ____ They are important sources of dietary fiber and many nutrients, including folic acid and vitamin C.

12. ____ Half of a person's plate should consist of choices from these two groups.

13. ____ At least half of all of these consumed should be "whole."

14. ____ One subgroup of these contains bran, germ, and endosperm.

15. ____ These products contain calcium, potassium, vitamin D, and protein.

16. ____ Within this group, dark green, red, and orange types have the best nutritional content.

17. ____ Animal sources of this include meat, poultry, seafood, and eggs.

Multiple Choice

18. MyPlate's guidelines state that half of a person's plate should be made up of
(A) Grains and protein
(B) Vegetables and fruits
(C) Seafood and dairy
(D) Grains and dairy

19. Vegetables that are this color have the best nutritional content:
(A) Dark green
(B) Light yellow
(C) Dark purple
(D) Light brown

20. Most of a person's fruit choices should be
(A) Frozen fruit
(B) Smoothies
(C) Cut-up fruit
(D) Fruit juice

21. What kinds of grains are best to consume?
(A) Refined grains
(B) White grains
(C) Whole grains
(D) Corn grains

22. Which of the following is considered a plant-based protein?
(A) Salmon
(B) Eggs
(C) Sausage
(D) Beans

23. Oatmeal and pasta are examples of foods made from which food group?
(A) Vegetables
(B) Fruits
(C) Grains
(D) Protein

24. Most dairy group choices should be
(A) Whole-fat
(B) 2% fat
(C) Half-and-half
(D) 1% fat

25. Which of the following foods is considered high in sodium?
(A) Apple
(B) Pickle
(C) Avocado
(D) Corn

3. Identify ways to assist clients in maintaining fluid balance

True or False

1. ____ Ice chips should be offered when a client has a swallowing problem.

2. ____ Fluid overload occurs when the body is unable to handle the amount of fluid consumed.

3. ____ The sense of thirst often diminishes in elderly people.

4. ____ People can become dehydrated by vomiting too much.

5. ____ If a client has an NPO order, he can drink water but no other type of fluid.

6. ____ In general the HHA should encourage clients to drink every time she sees them to help prevent dehydration.

7. ____ One symptom of dehydration is dark urine.

4. Identify nutritional problems of clients who are elderly or ill

Crossword

Across

4. Type of tube placed into the stomach through the abdominal wall for feeding a person (abbreviation)
5. Type of liquid that may be used for someone who has difficulty swallowing

Down

1. Skin breakdown due to weight loss can lead to these
2. Position clients should be in for eating
3. Temperature of food that may be preferable for someone suffering from nausea

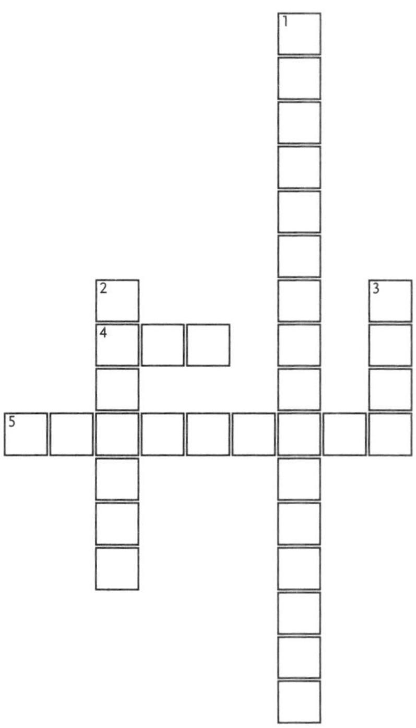

Short Answer

Make a check mark (✓) by all of the correct guidelines for working with clients who require tube feedings.

6. ____ The HHA should remove the tube when the feeding is finished.

7. ____ During the feeding, the client should remain in a sitting position with the head of the bed elevated at least 45 degrees.

8. ____ Discoloration or drainage around the opening should be reported.

9. ____ HHAs are responsible for slowly pouring feedings into the tube.

10. ____ HHAs should give careful skin care for clients who must remain in bed for long periods to help prevent pressure injuries.

11. ____ It is important for the HHA to wash their hands before assisting in any way with a tube feeding.

12. ____ After a client has had a tube feeding, the HHA should help the client to lie down flat on his back.

5. Demonstrate awareness of regional, cultural, and religious food preferences

Short Answer

Briefly describe some of the foods you ate while growing up. Were there any special dishes that your family made that were related to your culture, religion, or region?

____

____

____

____

____

____

____

____

Name: ______________________

____

____

____

6. List and define common health claims on food labels

Fill in the Blank

1. ______________________ meat, poultry, eggs, and dairy products come from animals that are given no antibiotics or growth hormones.

2. __________-__________ products may contain artificial sweeteners, such as saccharin or aspartame.

3. If a product is labeled __________-__________ or ______________________, it usually does not contain much fat.

4. Claims of ______________________, *healthy*, or *good for you* may have little or no meaning.

5. Clients who must reduce their sodium or salt intake should eat foods labeled __________-__________, __________ ______-__________, or __________-__________.

6. The best way to limit ______________________ is to avoid foods containing animal fats.

7. If a product is labeled __________ __________, it means that the chickens producing the eggs have been allowed access to the outside for an unspecified period of time.

8. For a product to be labeled __________-__________, gluten must be limited to less than 20 parts per million (ppm), and it should not contain any wheat, rye, barley, or crossbreeds of these grains.

7. Explain the information on the FDA-required Nutrition Facts label

Multiple Choice

1. Why does the label have a subcategory of *added sugars* under *total sugars*?
   (A) Because most people do not get enough sugar in their diet
   (B) Because added sugar is healthier than the sugar that a product naturally contains
   (C) Because it gives a suggestion for how much sugar to add to a food to make it sweeter
   (D) Because excessive sugar may be linked to a variety of diseases, and this helps people understand how much sugar has been added to a product

2. Which of the following minerals is required to be on the Nutrition Facts label?
   (A) Zinc
   (B) Selenium
   (C) Phosphate
   (D) Iron

3. The standardized nutrition label on all packaged foods is called the
   (A) Percentage label
   (B) Food Information label
   (C) Nutrition Facts label
   (D) Serving Size Information label

4. The recommended daily totals on the label are based on a __________-calorie diet.
   (A) 2,500
   (B) 2,000
   (C) 1,000
   (D) 5,000

8. Explain special diets

Matching

For each of the following diets, choose the best description from those listed below. Use each letter only once.

1. _____ Bland Diet
2. _____ Diabetic Diet
3. _____ Flexitarian Diet

4. _____ Fluid-Restricted Diet
5. _____ Gluten-Free Diet
6. _____ High-Potassium Diet
7. _____ High-Residue Diet
8. _____ Liquid Diet
9. _____ Low-Fat Diet
10. _____ Low-Protein Diet
11. _____ Low-Residue Diet
12. _____ Low-Sodium Diet
13. _____ Mechanical Soft Diet
14. _____ Modified-Calorie Diet
15. _____ Pescatarian Diet
16. _____ Pureed Diet
17. _____ Soft Diet
18. _____ Vegan Diet
19. _____ Vegetarian Diet

(A) To prevent further heart or kidney damage, doctors may restrict fluid intake on this diet.

(B) This diet consists of foods that are in a liquid state at body temperature, and it is usually ordered as *clear* or *full*.

(C) This diet consists of soft or chopped foods that are easy to chew; foods that are hard to chew and swallow, such as raw vegetables, are restricted.

(D) People who have kidney disease may also be on this diet, which encourages foods like vegetables, breads, and pasta.

(E) People who have had heart attacks or who have heart disease may be placed on this diet, which at a minimum limits the intake of saturated fat.

(F) Carb counting may be part of this diet, as the amount of carbohydrates eaten must be carefully regulated.

(G) Salt is restricted in this diet.

(H) This diet is used for losing weight or preventing weight gain.

(I) The food used in this diet has been ground into a thick paste of baby food consistency.

(J) Often used for people who have gastric ulcers, this diet involves avoiding alcohol, spicy foods, and citrus juices, among other items.

(K) Health reasons, a dislike of meat, a compassion for animals, or a belief in nonviolence may lead a person to this diet.

(L) Used for people with celiac disease, this diet eliminates foods containing wheat flour, such as tortillas, crackers, breads, and pasta.

(M) Foods high in this mineral will be encouraged in this diet; this includes bananas, prunes, dried apricots, figs, and sweet potatoes.

(N) This diet increases the amount of fiber and whole grains ingested and it helps prevent constipation.

(O) This is a completely plant-based diet that eliminates all animals, eggs, dairy products, and foods derived from animals.

(P) This diet is used for people who have bowel disorders and reduces the amount of fiber, whole grains, and raw fruits and vegetables ingested.

(Q) Plant-based foods are eaten primarily in this diet, but meats and other animal products are also eaten occasionally.

(R) Foods in this diet are chopped or blended and are prepared using blenders, food processors, meat grinders, or cutting utensils.

(S) All meats and poultry are eliminated in this diet, but fish and other seafood are allowed.

9. Describe guidelines for assisting with eating

Multiple Choice

1. In which position should clients be when they are eating?
   (A) Sitting upright
   (B) Reclining
   (C) Lying on their sides
   (D) Standing

2. Ways to promote a client's dignity while feeding include
   (A) Asking the client, "Can you eat quickly tonight? I've still got to give you a bath."
   (B) Asking the client, "Which food would you like to try first?"
   (C) Looking around the room while he is eating
   (D) Mixing food whether or not the client has requested it

3. What is the best way for the HHA to test the temperature of her client's food?
   (A) The HHA should touch the food before serving it.
   (B) The HHA should put the food in the freezer for a few minutes until the steam is gone.
   (C) The HHA should try a bite before the client does.
   (D) The HHA should put her hand over the dish to sense its heat.

True or False

4. ____ Clients who must be fed are often embarrassed and depressed about their dependence on another person.

5. ____ It is a good idea for the HHA to alternate offering food and drink while helping a client eat.

6. ____ The HHA should stand while helping a client eat.

7. ____ The HHA should give the client her full attention while the client is eating.

8. ____ The client's mouth should be empty before the HHA offers another bite of food.

9. ____ The HHA should refer to pureed green beans as "green stuff" so the client knows which dish the HHA is talking about.

10. Describe eating and swallowing problems a client may have

Multiple Choice

1. In order to prevent aspiration, the HHA should keep the client in the ________ position after eating for at least 30 minutes.
   (A) Upright
   (B) Reclining
   (C) Lying flat
   (D) Side

2. Which consistency refers to the thickness of a thick juice, which is able to be drunk from a cup?
   (A) Honey
   (B) Pudding
   (C) Pear
   (D) Nectar

3. The medical term for difficulty swallowing is
   (A) Aspiration
   (B) Dysphagia
   (C) Edema
   (D) Dyspnea

4. If a client has a doctor's order for thickened liquids, which of the following can the HHA offer to the client?
   (A) Water
   (B) Thickened soup
   (C) Broth
   (D) Milk

5. The International Dysphagia Diet Standardisation Initiative (IDDSI) created a framework with the goal of making these descriptions standard in all care settings:
   (A) Drink thicknesses only
   (B) Food textures only
   (C) Drink thicknesses and food textures
   (D) Foods and drinks allowed on various special diets

23

Meal Planning, Shopping, Preparation, and Storage

1. Explain how to prepare a basic food plan and list food shopping guidelines

Short Answer

Make a basic food plan for Monday through Friday. Include breakfast, lunch, dinner, and snacks.

MONDAY

Breakfast

Snack

Lunch

Snack

Dinner

Snack

TUESDAY

Breakfast

Snack

Lunch

Snack

Dinner

Snack

WEDNESDAY

Breakfast

Snack

Lunch

Snack

Dinner

Snack

THURSDAY

Breakfast

Snack

Lunch

Snack

Dinner

Snack

Name: ______________________

FRIDAY

Breakfast

Snack

Lunch

Snack

Dinner

Snack

Fill in the Blank

1. Avoid overly ______________________, already-mixed, or ready-made foods because they are more expensive and less nutritious.
2. Read ______________________ for ingredients that may be harmful to a client, such as excessive salt.
3. Estimate the ______________________ per serving by dividing the total cost by the number of servings.
4. For clients on a low-fat diet, take the ______________________ off chicken and turkey parts.
5. Buy fresh foods that are in season when they are at their ______________________ flavor.
6. Large amounts or larger sizes are usually more ______________________.
7. Cheaper cuts of meat tend to have more ______________________ in bones and fat.

Short Answer

8. List four factors to consider when buying food for clients.

____

____

____

____

____

9. Do you buy any organic and/or locally grown foods? If so, why is that important to you?

____

____

____

____

____

2. List guidelines for safe food preparation

Complete the Sentence

1. An HHA should wash hands *only before starting* | *before starting and frequently during* food preparation.
2. Sponges should be washed in the *washing machine* | *dishwasher* to disinfect them.
3. Frozen foods are best defrosted *in the refrigerator* | *on the counter.*
4. Perishable food should not be left out for longer than *30 minutes* | *2 hours.*
5. Poultry needs to be cooked *thoroughly* | *to at least medium rare* to kill microorganisms.
6. If an HHA sneezes during food preparation, they should *call in sick for the rest of the shift* | *wash hands immediately.*
7. It is best to use separate cutting boards for *sweet and savory foods* | *meats and vegetables.*
8. After a knife has been used to cut meat, it must be *washed in hot, soapy water* | *soaked in bleach* and allowed to air-dry.
9. If a person has a weakened immune system because of cancer, a foodborne illness can *strengthen the immune system* | *be dangerous and even deadly.*

10. Elderly people are at increased risk for foodborne illnesses because they *often have reduced appetites | often have diminished senses and may not know food is spoiled.*

3. Identify methods of food preparation

Matching

For each method of food preparation, identify the correct description. Use each letter only once.

1. _____ Baking
2. _____ Boiling
3. _____ Braising
4. _____ Broiling
5. _____ Frying
6. _____ Microwaving
7. _____ Poaching
8. _____ Roasting
9. _____ Sautéing
10. _____ Steaming

(A) Safe for defrosting, reheating, and cooking, but this method can cause cold spots.

(B) Cooked in barely boiling water or other liquids; this is an ideal way to prepare fish and eggs.

(C) Used for meats, poultry, and some vegetables, this method may involve mixing items with oils or spices before cooking and basting meats or poultry during cooking.

(D) The best method for cooking pasta, noodles, and rice

(E) Used in an oven at moderate heat, this method is appropriate for many foods such as breads, fish, vegetables, and casseroles.

(F) A quick way to cook vegetables and meats by using a small amount of oil in a frying pan and stirring constantly

(G) A small amount of water is boiled in the bottom of a saucepan, and food is set over it in a basket or colander.

(H) The least healthy way to cook, this method uses a lot of fat.

(I) This method can be used to melt cheese or brown the top of a casserole.

(J) A slow-cooking method that uses moist heat to cook meat or vegetables at a temperature just below boiling

4. Identify four methods of low-fat food preparation

Fill in the Blank

1. ______________________________ allows fats in meat to drip out before food is consumed, which lowers fat content.
2. Plan meals around ______________________________ or ______________________________ to help cut out the fat content.
3. Sometimes high-fat ingredients can be ______________ ______________ or replaced to lower the fat content of a recipe.
4. ______________________________ meat on paper towels after you brown it.
5. Leave out ______________________________ on sandwiches or on top of casseroles.
6. An example of a low-fat meal based on vegetables and grains is beans and ______________________________.
7. Boiling, steaming, broiling, roasting, and ______________________________ are all methods of cooking that require little fat.
8. Try substituting ____________ ____________ ____________ for mayonnaise or sour cream.
9. For people who follow a vegan diet, ______________-______________ foods can be substituted for cheese and cream.

Name: ______________________________

5. List four guidelines for safe food storage

Multiple Choice

1. After shopping, which of the following foods should be put away first?
   (A) Crackers
   (B) Milk
   (C) Pasta
   (D) Cereal

2. It is a good idea to keep easily spoiled items in the
   (A) Door of the refrigerator
   (B) Cupboard
   (C) Rear of the refrigerator
   (D) Pantry

3. Refrigerator temperature should be between
   (A) 0°F and 10°F
   (B) 36°F and 40°F
   (C) 10°F and 20°F
   (D) 62°F and 66°F

4. Food should not be left out for more than ________ hours.
   (A) 5
   (B) 3
   (C) 2
   (D) 12

5. If the HHA is not sure whether food is spoiled, she should
   (A) Discard it
   (B) Serve it and see if anyone complains or feels ill
   (C) Cook it for a longer time than usual
   (D) Smell it after cooking it to be sure it is safe

6. Food that can be composted includes
   (A) Canola oil
   (B) Fish bones
   (C) Yogurt
   (D) Coffee grounds

24

Managing Time, Energy, and Money

1. Explain ways to work more efficiently

Short Answer

1. Give at least one example each (other than what is in the book) of how you can distribute tasks, prioritize tasks, and simplify tasks while working as an HHA.

2. List five ways to conserve time and energy.

2. Describe how to follow an established work plan with the client and family

Short Answer

Pick the busiest day you will have next week, and draft a work plan for that day. List tasks to complete and prioritize them.

Name: ____________________

3. Discuss ways to handle inappropriate requests

Short Answer

Read the following scenario and answer the question.

Richard, an HHA, is preparing to leave his client's home for the day. Mr. Perez, his client, demands that Richard buy him some soup at the grocery store before he leaves. This errand is not in the care plan, but Mr. Perez tells him that he really wants some soup. Mr. Perez begins to cry. What should Richard do in this situation?

____

4. List five money-saving homemaking tips

Short Answer

List and briefly explain five money-saving tips.

____

5. List guidelines for handling a client's money

Short Answer

1. What are your state's guidelines for handling a client's money?

____

True or False

2. ____ It is fine for an HHA to use her client's money for her own things as long as she pays it back soon.
3. ____ The HHA should estimate the amount of money they will need before requesting it.
4. ____ The HHA should return receipts to the client or family member as soon as possible.
5. ____ The HHA should keep a client's cash separate from her own.
6. ____ If a client is unsure about his budget, the HHA should give him financial advice and budgeting tips.

25

Caring for Yourself and Your Career

1. Discuss different types of careers in the healthcare field

True or False

1. ____ Direct service workers include salespeople, waiters, and bartenders.
2. ____ X-ray technicians work in diagnostic services.
3. ____ Receptionists, office managers, and billing staff are considered part of the healthcare field.
4. ____ Health educators have job opportunities within the healthcare field.
5. ____ Counselors and social workers are not part of the healthcare field.

2. Explain how to find a job

Short Answer

List three resources you should try when looking for potential employers.

____

____

____

____

____

____

____

____

3. Identify documents that may be required when applying for a job and explain how to write a résumé

Short Answer

1. List four documents that may be needed when applying for a job.

____

____

____

____

____

Complete the Sentence

2. *Friends and relatives* | *Former employers or teachers* are the best references to use for a potential job.
3. Ideally, a person's résumé should fit on *one page of paper* | *an index card.*
4. A résumé should include a list of the person's *religious and political beliefs* | *educational experience.*
5. Employers *must have* | *generally prefer to have* files showing that all employees are legally allowed to work in this country.
6. A cover letter should emphasize the skills a person has that *are not common among their peers* | *make them a good match for the position.*

Name: ______________________________

4. Demonstrate completing an effective job application

Short Answer

Complete the sample job application.

Employment Application

Personal Information	
Name:	Date:
Home Address:	
City, State, Zip:	
Email Address:	
Home Phone:	Business Phone:
US Citizen?	If Not, Give Visa No. and Expiration Date:

Position Applying For	
Title:	Salary Desired:
Referred By:	Date Available:

Education	
High School (Name, City, State):	
Graduation Date:	
Technical or Undergraduate School:	
Dates Attended:	Degree Major:

References

5. Demonstrate competence in job interview techniques

Short Answer

Make a check mark (✓) next to the actions appropriate for job interviews.

1. ____ Wearing jeans
2. ____ Looking happy to be there
3. ____ Asking if it is okay to smoke during the interview
4. ____ Wearing very little jewelry
5. ____ Asking how many hours you would work
6. ____ Bringing your child with you if you cannot find a babysitter
7. ____ Wearing your nicest perfume
8. ____ Sitting up straight
9. ____ Asking what benefits the employer offers
10. ____ Shaking hands with interviewer
11. ____ Eating a granola bar during the interview
12. ____ Asking if you got the job at the end of the interview
13. ____ Letting the interviewer know some of the negative things your former boss did
14. ____ Asking how soon a decision about the position will be made

6. Discuss appropriate responses to feedback

Short Answer

Read the following and mark whether they are examples of constructive feedback or hostile criticism. Use a C *for constructive and an* H *for hostile.*

1. ____ "You are a horrible person."
2. ____ "If you weren't so slow, things might get done around here."
3. ____ "Some of your reports are not complete; try to be more accurate."

4. ____ "That was the worst meal I've ever eaten."

5. ____ "I'm not sure that you understood what I meant. Let me rephrase the issue."

6. ____ "Where did you learn how to clean?"

7. ____ "That was a stupid idea."

8. ____ "That procedure could have been performed in a more efficient way."

9. ____ "Try to make more of an effort to listen carefully."

10. ____ "Stop being so lazy."

7. Identify effective ways to make a complaint to an employer or supervisor and discuss how to manage conflict

Short Answer

Read the following scenario and answer the question.

Anne is an HHA who works 3 days a week for her client, Mrs. Singer. Generally, Mrs. Singer's son, Benjamin, is there as well, and he and Anne work as a team. Benjamin finds a new job and cannot be home during the day anymore. The next time Anne arrives, Mrs. Singer is moody and distant. She is reluctant to follow the care plan, and she tells Anne that she will not take a bath until Benjamin comes home. She also refuses to eat food that Anne has cooked, insisting she can only eat her son's cooking. After some gentle urging, Anne gets Mrs. Singer to eat and take a bath.

The next time Anne works, Mrs. Singer drops her plate on the floor and tells Anne that she is a lousy cook. She tells her to fix a new meal and clean up the mess. Anne does both although she feels very upset.

1. Should this be reported to a supervisor? If so, how should it be reported?

____

____

____

____

____

____

____

____

____

____

____

____

____

____

Multiple Choice

2. When is an appropriate time to discuss an issue that is causing conflict in the workplace?
   (A) When the HHA decides she cannot take it anymore
   (B) When the HHA is upset because something has just occurred
   (C) Right before the HHA gives her notice
   (D) When the supervisor has decided on a proper time and place

3. When trying to resolve a conflict, the HHA should
   (A) Interrupt the other person if the HHA might forget what she is going to say
   (B) Sit back in the chair with her arms crossed over her chest
   (C) Take turns speaking
   (D) Yell at the other person if it seems like her point is not understood

4. When discussing conflict, the HHA should
   (A) State how she feels when a behavior occurs
   (B) Name-call
   (C) Not look the other person in the eye
   (D) Keep the TV on to fill awkward silences

Name: ____________________

5. To resolve a conflict, the HHA should be prepared to
   (A) Compromise
   (B) Quit
   (C) Argue
   (D) Interrupt

8. Identify guidelines for making job changes

Fill in the Blank

1. The HHA should always give an employer ____________________ weeks' written notice that he will be leaving.
2. Potential future employers may talk with the HHA's past ____________________.
3. If an HHA decides to change jobs, he should be ____________________.

9. List your state's requirements for maintaining certification

Short Answer

1. How many hours of in-service education are required each year by your state?

2. How long is an absence from working allowed, without retraining, in your state?

10. Describe continuing education for home health aides

True or False

1. ____ The federal government requires 20 hours of continuing education each year.
2. ____ Regulations regarding care can change.
3. ____ States require less continuing education than the federal government.
4. ____ In-service continuing education courses help keep knowledge fresh.

Short Answer

5. List three of the responsibilities an HHA has regarding continuing education.

11. Define *stress* and *stressor* and list examples

Short Answer

What are some situations that make you experience stress? How do you react when you are stressed?

12. Explain ways to manage stress

Multiple Choice

1. Stress is a(n) ______________ response.
   (A) Rare
   (B) Physical and emotional
   (C) Anti-inflammatory
   (D) Antibody
2. When the heart beats fast in stressful situations, it can be a result of an increase of the hormone
   (A) Testosterone
   (B) Estrogen
   (C) Adrenaline
   (D) Progesterone
3. A healthy lifestyle includes
   (A) Eating when a person is not hungry to calm down
   (B) Exercising regularly
   (C) Smoking a few cigarettes a week
   (D) Complaining about a job
4. Which of the following is a sign that a person is not managing stress?
   (A) Preparing meals ahead of time
   (B) Taking deep breaths and relaxing
   (C) Feeling alert and positive
   (D) Not being able to focus on work
5. Which of the following are appropriate people for an HHA to turn to for help in managing stress?
   (A) Clients
   (B) Supervisors
   (C) Clients' family members
   (D) Clients' friends

13. Demonstrate two effective relaxation techniques

Short Answer

Try one of the relaxation techniques listed on page 426 of the textbook. Describe how you felt after the experience.

14. Describe how to develop a personal stress management plan

Short Answer

Write out your own personal stress management plan. Be sure to include things like diet, exercise, relaxation exercises, entertainment, etc.

Name: ____________________

15. List five guidelines for managing time

Short Answer

Choose one of the five guidelines for managing time and describe how it could apply to your personal time and to your time on the job.

16. Demonstrate an understanding of the basics of money management

Short Answer

Choose one of the topics covered in this learning objective. How might a person reduce stress by managing money in that way?

17. Demonstrate an understanding that money matters are emotional

Short Answer

When was the last time you wanted something you could not afford? How did it make you feel? What did you do?

18. List ways to remind yourself that your work is important, valuable, and meaningful

Short Answer

1. List five things that you have learned in this course that have surprised or excited you.

2. List five things that you are looking forward to doing when you start working as an HHA.

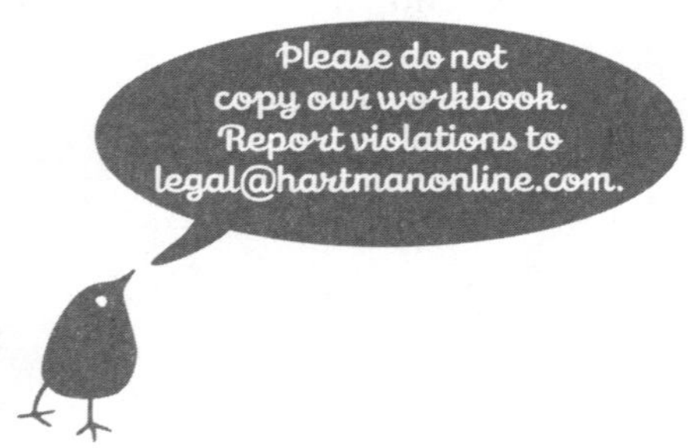

Name: ________________________________

Procedure Checklists

5
Infection Prevention and Standard Precautions

Washing hands (hand hygiene)			
		yes	no
1.	Turns on water at sink.		
2.	Wets hands and wrists thoroughly.		
3.	Applies soap to hands.		
4.	Keeps hands lower than elbows and fingertips down. Rubs hands together and lathers all surfaces of wrists, hands, and fingers, using friction for at least 20 seconds.		
5.	Cleans nails by rubbing them in palm of other hand.		
6.	Keeps hands lower than elbows and fingertips down. Without touching sink, rinses all surfaces of wrists and hands, running water from wrists to fingertips.		
7.	Uses clean, dry paper towel to dry all surfaces of fingers, hands, and wrists. Discards towel without touching container.		
8.	Uses clean, dry paper towel to turn off faucet and discards towel without contaminating hands.		

Date Reviewed ____________ Instructor Signature ____________

Date Performed ____________ Instructor Signature ____________

Putting on (donning) and removing (doffing) a gown			
		yes	no
1.	Washes hands.		
2.	Opens gown and allows it to unfold without shaking it or touching it to the floor. Places arms through each sleeve.		
3.	Fastens neck opening and pulls gown until it completely covers clothing. Secures gown at waist.		
4.	Puts on gloves after putting on gown.		
5.	When removing gown, removes and discards gloves first. Then unfastens gown at neck and waist.		
6.	Removes gown without touching the outside of gown. Rolls dirty side in while holding gown away from body. Discards gown. Washes hands.		

Date Reviewed ____________ Instructor Signature ____________

Date Performed ____________ Instructor Signature ____________

Putting on (donning) a mask and goggles			
		yes	no
1.	Washes hands.		
2.	For a respirator, holds mask in cupped hand with top end at fingertips. For other mask, picks up mask by top strings or elastic strap. Does not touch mask where it touches face.		

Name: ______________________

		yes	no
3.	For a respirator, pulls elastic straps over head, placing top strap on the crown of the head and bottom strap at the base of the neck without crisscrossing straps. For a mask with strings, ties top strings first, then bottom strings. For a mask with loops, hooks loops securely behind ears.		
4.	Pinches the metal strip at the top of the mask tightly around nose. Fits mask snugly around face and below chin. For a respirator, performs user seal check as trained.		
5.	Puts on goggles.		
6.	Puts on gloves.		

Date Reviewed ______ Instructor Signature ______

Date Performed ______ Instructor Signature ______

Putting on (donning) gloves

		yes	no
1.	Washes hands.		
2.	If right-handed, slides one glove on left hand (reverses if left-handed).		
3.	With gloved hand, slides other hand into the second glove.		
4.	Interlaces fingers to smooth out folds and create a comfortable fit.		
5.	Carefully checks for tears, holes, cracks, or spots. Replaces glove if needed.		
6.	Adjusts gloves for correct fit. If wearing a gown, pulls the cuff of the gloves over sleeves of gown.		

Date Reviewed ______ Instructor Signature ______

Date Performed ______ Instructor Signature ______

Removing (doffing) gloves

		yes	no
1.	Touches only the outside of one glove and grasps the other glove at the palm, pulling glove off.		
2.	With ungloved hand, slips two fingers underneath cuff of remaining glove. Does not touch any part of the outside of glove.		
3.	Pulls down, turning glove inside out and over the first glove. One glove from its clean inner side should be holding the other glove inside it.		
4.	Discards gloves.		
5.	Washes hands.		

Date Reviewed ______ Instructor Signature ______

Date Performed ______ Instructor Signature ______

Donning a full set of PPE

		yes	no
1.	Washes hands.		
2.	Puts on gown properly.		
3.	Puts on mask or respirator properly.		
4.	Puts on goggles or face shield properly.		
5.	Puts on gloves properly.		

Date Reviewed ______ Instructor Signature ______

Date Performed ______ Instructor Signature ______

Doffing a full set of PPE

		yes	no
1.	Removes and discards gloves properly.		
2.	Removes and discards goggles or face shield properly.		

3.	Removes and discards gown properly.		
4.	Removes and discards mask properly.		
5.	Washes hands.		

Date Reviewed ______ Instructor Signature ______

Date Performed ______ Instructor Signature ______

Disinfecting using wet heat

		yes	no
1.	Washes hands.		
2.	Places items in the pot and fills it with water, covering all items.		
3.	Places lid on pot and places pot on stove.		
4.	Brings water to a boil. Boils items for 20 minutes.		
5.	Turns off heat. Allows items and water to cool.		
6.	After items have cooled, removes cover and then items. Places items on rack or towel to dry.		
7.	Washes and dries equipment. Returns to proper storage.		
8.	Washes hands.		
9.	Documents procedure.		

Date Reviewed ______ Instructor Signature ______

Date Performed ______ Instructor Signature ______

Disinfecting using dry heat

		yes	no
1.	Washes hands.		
2.	Places items in the pan and places pan or sheet in oven.		
3.	Turns on oven to 350°F and bakes items for 1 hour.		
4.	Turns off heat. Allows items to cool.		
5.	After items have cooled, removes items.		
6.	Stores items.		
7.	Washes and dries equipment. Returns to proper storage.		
8.	Washes hands.		
9.	Documents procedure.		

Date Reviewed ______ Instructor Signature ______

Date Performed ______ Instructor Signature ______

7
Emergency Care and Disaster Preparation

Performing abdominal thrusts for the conscious person

		yes	no
1.	Stands behind person and brings arms under person's arms. Wraps arms around person's waist.		
2.	Makes a fist with one hand. Places flat, thumb side of the fist against person's abdomen, above the navel but below the breastbone.		
3.	Grasps the fist with other hand. Pulls both hands toward self and up, quickly and forcefully.		
4.	Repeats until object is pushed out or person loses consciousness.		
5.	Reports and documents incident.		

Date Reviewed ______ Instructor Signature ______

Date Performed ______ Instructor Signature ______

Name: ______________________

Clearing an obstructed airway in a conscious infant		yes	no
1.	Lays the infant face down on forearm; if sitting, rests the arm holding the infant's torso on lap or thigh. Supports infant's jaw and head with hand.		
2.	Delivers up to five back blows.		
3.	If the obstruction is not expelled, turns infant onto his back while supporting the head. Delivers up to five chest thrusts.		
4.	Repeats, alternating five back blows and five chest thrusts until object is pushed out or infant loses consciousness.		
5.	Reports and documents incident.		

Date Reviewed ______ Instructor Signature ______

Date Performed ______ Instructor Signature ______

Responding to shock		yes	no
1.	Calls for help immediately.		
2.	Puts on gloves and controls bleeding if necessary.		
3.	Has the person lie down on her back unless bleeding from the mouth or vomiting. Elevates the legs unless person has a head, neck, back, spinal, or abdominal injury; breathing difficulties; or fractures.		
4.	Checks pulse and respirations if possible. Begins CPR (as trained and allowed) if breathing and pulse are absent.		
5.	Keeps person as calm and comfortable as possible.		
6.	Maintains normal body temperature.		
7.	Does not give person food or liquids.		
8.	Reports and documents incident.		

Date Reviewed ______ Instructor Signature ______

Date Performed ______ Instructor Signature ______

Responding to a myocardial infarction		yes	no
1.	Calls for help immediately.		
2.	Places person in a comfortable position. Encourages him to rest, and reassures him that he will not be left alone.		
3.	Loosens clothing around the neck.		
4.	Does not give person food or liquids.		
5.	Monitors person's breathing and pulse. Begins CPR (as trained and allowed) if breathing and pulse are absent.		
6.	Stays with person until help arrives.		
7.	Reports and documents incident.		

Date Reviewed ______ Instructor Signature ______

Date Performed ______ Instructor Signature ______

Controlling bleeding		yes	no
1.	Calls for help immediately.		
2.	Puts on gloves.		
3.	Holds thick sterile pad, clean cloth, or clean towel against the wound.		

		yes	no
4.	Presses down hard directly on the bleeding wound until help arrives. Does not decrease pressure. Puts additional pads over the first pad if blood seeps through. Does not remove the first pad.		
5.	Raises the wound above level of the heart to slow bleeding.		
6.	When bleeding is under control, secures dressing to keep it in place. Checks person for symptoms of shock. Stays with person until help arrives.		
7.	Removes and discards gloves. Washes hands.		
8.	Reports and documents incident.		

Date Reviewed ____________ Instructor Signature ____________

Date Performed ____________ Instructor Signature ____________

Treating burns

		yes	no
	Minor burns:		
1.	Puts on gloves.		
2.	Uses cool, clean water (not ice or ice water) to decrease the skin temperature and prevent further injury. Does not use ointment, salve, or grease. Dampens a clean cloth with cool water and covers burn.		
3.	Covers area with a dry, clean dressing or nonadhesive sterile bandage.		
4.	Removes and discards gloves. Washes hands.		
5.	Reports and documents incident.		
	Serious burns:		
1.	Removes person from source of the burn.		
2.	Calls for help immediately. Puts on gloves.		
3.	Checks for breathing, pulse, and severe bleeding. Begins CPR (as trained and allowed) if breathing and pulse are absent. Does not apply ointment, water, salve, or grease.		
4.	Does not remove clothing from burned areas. Covers burn with sterile gauze or a clean sheet without rubbing skin.		
5.	Does not give person food or liquids.		
6.	Monitors vital signs and waits for emergency medical help.		
7.	Removes and discards gloves. Washes hands.		
8.	Reports and documents incident.		

Date Reviewed ____________ Instructor Signature ____________

Date Performed ____________ Instructor Signature ____________

Responding to seizures

		yes	no
1.	Notes the time. Puts on gloves.		
2.	Lowers person to the floor.		
3.	Has someone call emergency medical help. Does not leave person unless has to get medical help.		
4.	Moves furniture away to prevent injury.		
5.	Does not try to restrain the person or stop the seizure.		
6.	Does not force anything between the person's teeth. Does not place hands in the person's mouth.		
7.	Does not give food or fluids.		

Name: ______________________

		yes	no
8.	When the seizure is over, notes time. Turns person to left side if head, neck, back, spinal, or abdominal injuries are not suspected. Checks breathing and pulse. Begins CPR (as trained and allowed) if breathing and pulse are absent.		
9.	Removes and discards gloves. Washes hands.		
10.	Reports and documents incident.		

Date Reviewed ______ Instructor Signature ______

Date Performed ______ Instructor Signature ______

Responding to fainting

		yes	no
1.	Has person lie down or sit down before fainting occurs.		
2.	If person is sitting, has him bend forward. If person is lying flat on his back and there are no head, neck, back, spinal, or abdominal injuries; breathing difficulties; or fractures, elevates his legs about 12 inches.		
3.	Loosens any tight clothing.		
4.	Has person stay in position for at least 5 minutes after symptoms disappear.		
5.	Helps person get up slowly. Continues to observe him for symptoms of fainting.		
6.	If person faints, lowers him to floor, positioning him on his back. Elevates legs 12 inches if no head, neck, back, spinal, or abdominal injuries are suspected. Contacts supervisor.		

		yes	no
7.	Reports and documents incident.		

Date Reviewed ______ Instructor Signature ______

Date Performed ______ Instructor Signature ______

Responding to a nosebleed

		yes	no
1.	Elevates head of the bed or tells client to remain in sitting position, leaning forward. Offers tissues or a clean cloth.		
2.	Puts on gloves. Applies firm pressure on both sides of the nose, near the bridge. Squeezes sides with thumb and forefinger.		
3.	Applies pressure consistently until bleeding stops.		
4.	Uses a cool cloth or ice wrapped in a cloth on bridge of nose to slow blood flow.		
5.	Removes and discards gloves. Washes hands.		
6.	Reports and documents incident.		

Date Reviewed ______ Instructor Signature ______

Date Performed ______ Instructor Signature ______

Helping a client who has fallen

		yes	no
1.	Assesses client's condition and gets help if condition warrants it.		
2.	Looks for broken bones.		
3.	Asks client to move each body part separately to observe.		
4.	***If sprain or fracture is suspected:*** Calls supervisor and reports fall.		
	Keeps injured area in one position. Does not move client.		

Name: ______________________________

	Keeps client covered with blanket.		
	If no injury is suspected: Makes client comfortable.		
	Calls supervisor and reports fall.		
	Does not move client until supervisor has been contacted.		
5.	Reports and documents incident.		

Date Reviewed ______ Instructor Signature ______

Date Performed ______ Instructor Signature ______

9
Body Systems and Related Conditions

Providing foot care for a client with diabetes

		yes	no
1.	Washes hands.		
2.	Explains procedure to client, speaking clearly, slowly, and directly. Maintains face-to-face contact whenever possible.		
3.	Provides privacy.		
4.	Fills the basin halfway with warm water. Tests water temperature and has client check water temperature. Adjusts if necessary.		
5.	Places basin on bath mat or towel in a comfortable position for client. Supports foot and ankle throughout.		
6.	Puts on gloves.		
7.	Removes socks and submerges feet. Soaks for 15 to 20 minutes.		
8.	Washes feet one at a time. Rinses the feet.		
9.	Pats the feet dry, including between the toes.		
10.	Gently rubs lotion into the feet with circular strokes. Does not put lotion between the toes.		
11.	Observes the skin for signs of dryness, irritation, etc.		
12.	Helps client put on socks and shoes or slippers.		
13.	Puts used linens in laundry. Cleans and stores basin and supplies.		
14.	Removes and discards gloves. Washes hands.		
15.	Documents procedure and any observations.		

Date Reviewed ______ Instructor Signature ______

Date Performed ______ Instructor Signature ______

12
Positioning, Transfers, and Ambulation

Moving a client up in bed

		yes	no
1.	***If client cannot assist:*** Washes hands.		
2.	Explains procedure to client, speaking clearly, slowly, and directly. Maintains face-to-face contact whenever possible.		
3.	Provides privacy.		
4.	Adjusts bed to a safe working level. Locks bed wheels.		
5.	Lowers head of bed. Moves pillow to head of bed.		
6.	Stands behind head of bed with feet apart and one foot slightly in front of other.		
7.	Rolls and grasps top of draw sheet. Bends knees, keeping back straight, and rocks weight from front foot to back foot, while pulling client toward head of bed.		
8.	Positions client comfortably, arranges pillow and blankets, unrolls draw sheet and leaves in place, and returns bed to lowest position.		

Name: ______________________

9.	Washes hands.		
10.	Documents procedure and any observations.		

Date Reviewed ____________ Instructor Signature ____________

Date Reviewed ____________ Instructor Signature ____________

1.	***When help from another person is available:*** Washes hands.		
2.	Explains procedure to client, speaking clearly, slowly, and directly. Maintains face-to-face contact whenever possible.		
3.	Provides privacy.		
4.	Adjusts bed to a safe working level. Locks bed wheels.		
5.	Lowers head of bed. Moves pillow to head of bed.		
6.	Stands on opposite side of bed from helper. Faces head of bed and points foot closer to head of bed toward head of bed.		
7.	Rolls draw sheet up to client's side and grasps sheet, with one hand at client's shoulders and the other at client's hips.		
8.	Shifts weight to back foot and on count of 3, both workers shift weight to forward feet while sliding draw sheet and client toward head of bed.		
9.	Positions client comfortably, arranges pillow and blankets, unrolls draw sheet, and returns bed to lowest position.		
10.	Washes hands.		
11.	Documents procedure and any observations.		

Date Reviewed ____________ Instructor Signature ____________

Date Performed ____________ Instructor Signature ____________

Moving a client to the side of the bed

		yes	no
1.	Washes hands.		
2.	Explains procedure to client, speaking clearly, slowly, and directly. Maintains face-to-face contact whenever possible.		
3.	Provides privacy.		
4.	Adjusts bed to a safe working level. Locks bed wheels. Lowers head of bed.		
5.	Stands on same side of bed to which client will be moved.		
6.	***With a draw sheet:*** Rolls draw sheet up to client's side and grasps sheet, with one hand at client's shoulders and the other at client's hips. Places one knee against side of bed, leans back, and pulls draw sheet and client toward self on the count of 3. Unrolls draw sheet and leaves in place.		
	Without a draw sheet: Slides hands under client's head and shoulders and moves toward self. Slides hands under client's midsection and moves toward self. Slides hands under client's hips and legs and moves toward self.		
7.	Returns bed to lowest position.		
8.	Washes hands.		
9.	Documents procedure and any observations.		

Date Reviewed ____________ Instructor Signature ____________

Date Performed ____________ Instructor Signature ____________

Name: ____________________

Positioning a client on his side			
		yes	no
1.	Washes hands.		
2.	Explains procedure to client, speaking clearly, slowly, and directly. Maintains face-to-face contact whenever possible.		
3.	Provides privacy.		
4.	Adjusts bed to a safe working level. Locks bed wheels. Lowers head of bed.		
5.	Moves client toward side of bed nearest self. Raises far side rail.		
6.	***Turning a client away from self:*** Crosses client's arms over his chest and crosses his near leg over his far leg. Stands with feet apart and knees bent. Places one hand on client's near shoulder and the other hand on his near hip. Gently rolls client onto his side as one unit, toward the raised side rail.		
	Turning a client toward self: Crosses client's far arm over his chest and moves arm on side client is being turned to out of the way. Crosses his far leg over his near leg. Stands with feet apart and knees bent. Places one hand on client's far shoulder and the other hand on his far hip. Gently rolls client onto his side as one unit, toward self.		
7.	Positions client properly and comfortably, using pillows or other supports.		
8.	Returns bed to lowest position.		
9.	Washes hands.		
10.	Documents procedure and any observations.		

Date Reviewed ____________ Instructor Signature ____________

Date Performed ____________ Instructor Signature ____________

Logrolling a client			
		yes	no
1.	Washes hands.		
2.	Explains procedure to client, speaking clearly, slowly, and directly. Maintains face-to-face contact whenever possible.		
3.	Provides privacy.		
4.	Adjusts bed to a safe working level. Locks bed wheels. Lowers head of bed.		
5.	Both workers stand on same side of bed, one at the client's head and shoulders, one near the midsection.		
6.	Places pillow under the client's head. Places client's arm across his chest and places a pillow between his knees.		
7.	Stands with feet about shoulder-width apart, bends knees, and grasps draw sheet on far side.		
8.	Rolls client toward selves on count of 3, turning client as a unit.		
9.	Positions client comfortably, arranges pillow and blankets, checks for proper body alignment, unrolls draw sheet, and returns bed to lowest position.		
10.	Washes hands.		
11.	Documents procedure and any observations.		

Date Reviewed ____________ Instructor Signature ____________

Date Performed ____________ Instructor Signature ____________

Name: ________________________________

Assisting a client to sit up on the side of the bed: dangling

		yes	no
1.	Washes hands.		
2.	Explains procedure to client, speaking clearly, slowly, and directly. Maintains face-to-face contact whenever possible.		
3.	Provides privacy.		
4.	Adjusts the bed to lowest position. Locks bed wheels.		
5.	Raises head of bed to sitting position. Fanfolds top covers to foot of bed and assists client to turn onto side, facing self.		
6.	Has client reach across chest with top arm and place hand on edge of bed near opposite shoulder. Asks client to push down on that hand while swinging legs over the side of bed.		
7.	If client needs assistance, stands with legs shoulder-width apart and bends knees.		
8.	Places one arm under client's shoulder blades and the other under his thighs.		
9.	Turns client into sitting position on count of 3.		
10.	With client holding on to edge of mattress, puts nonskid shoes on client and fastens them. Has client dangle as long as directed. Does not leave client alone.		
11.	Returns client safely to bed after removing shoes, or completes walking or transfer according to care plan. Returns bed to lowest position.		
12.	Washes hands.		
13.	Documents procedure and any observations.		

Date Reviewed	Instructor Signature
Date Performed	Instructor Signature

Transferring a client from a bed to a wheelchair

		yes	no
1.	Washes hands.		
2.	Explains procedure to client, speaking clearly, slowly, and directly. Maintains face-to-face contact whenever possible.		
3.	Provides privacy.		
4.	Places wheelchair at the head of the bed, facing the foot of the bed, or at the foot of bed, facing the head of bed. Wheelchair should be on client's stronger side. Removes footrests. Locks wheelchair wheels.		
5.	Raises head of bed and adjusts bed level to lowest position. Locks bed wheels.		
6.	Assists client to sitting position with feet flat on floor. Lets client sit for a few minutes. Puts nonskid shoes on client and fastens them.		
7.	Stands in front of client with feet about shoulder-width apart. Bends knees. Places transfer belt around client's waist over clothing and grasps belt on both sides with hands in upward position.		
8.	Provides instructions to assist with transfer. Braces client's lower legs. Helps client stand on count of 3.		

Name: ______________________________

9.	Tells client to take small steps to the chair while turning his back toward chair. Helps client to pivot to front of chair if necessary.		
10.	Asks client to put hands on chair armrests and helps client to lower himself into the chair.		
11.	Attaches footrests and places client's feet on them. Positions client in the chair properly and removes transfer belt. Places robe over lap as needed.		
12.	Washes hands.		
13.	Documents procedure and any observations.		

_______________ Date Reviewed ______________________ Instructor Signature

_______________ Date Performed ______________________ Instructor Signature

Helping a client transfer using a slide board

		yes	no
1.	Washes hands.		
2.	Explains procedure to client, speaking clearly, slowly, and directly. Maintains face-to-face contact whenever possible.		
3.	Provides privacy.		
4.	Places wheelchair at the head of the bed, facing the foot of the bed, or at the foot of bed, facing the head of bed. Wheelchair should be on client's stronger side. Removes footrests. Locks wheelchair wheels.		
5.	Raises head of bed and adjusts bed level to lowest position. Locks bed wheels.		
6.	Assists client to sitting position with feet flat on floor. Lets client sit for a few minutes. Puts non-skid shoes on client and fastens them.		
7.	Has client lean away from the transfer side.		
8.	Places one end of slide board under client's buttocks and thighs and the other end on the surface to which client is transferring.		
9.	Instructs client to push up with hands and scoot across the board.		
10.	If client needs assistance, braces client's knees, grasps the transfer belt, and instructs client to lean forward. Helps client scoot across the board, without dragging client.		
11.	Removes slide board after transfer is complete. Positions client comfortably and safely.		
12.	Washes hands.		
13.	Documents procedure and any observations.		

_______________ Date Reviewed ______________________ Instructor Signature

_______________ Date Performed ______________________ Instructor Signature

Transferring a client using a mechanical lift

		yes	no
1.	Washes hands.		
2.	Explains procedure to client, speaking clearly, slowly, and directly. Maintains face-to-face contact whenever possible.		
3.	Provides privacy.		
4.	Locks bed wheels. Positions wheelchair next to bed and locks brakes.		
5.	Positions sling under client.		
6.	Positions mechanical lift next to bed, opening the base to its widest point; pushes base of lift under bed. Positions overhead bar directly over client.		

Name: ______________________

7.	Attaches straps to sling properly.		
8.	Raises client in sling 2 inches above bed. Pauses to let client gain balance.		
9.	Rolls mechanical lift to position client over chair or wheelchair. Lifting partner supports and guides client's body.		
10.	Slowly lowers client into chair or wheelchair, pushing down gently on client's knees.		
11.	Undoes straps from overhead bar to sling, leaving sling in place.		
12.	Positions client comfortably and correctly.		
13.	Washes hands.		
14.	Documents procedure and any observations.		

Date Reviewed ______ Instructor Signature ______

Date Performed ______ Instructor Signature ______

Assisting a client to ambulate

		yes	no
1.	Washes hands.		
2.	Explains procedure to client, speaking clearly, slowly, and directly. Maintains face-to-face contact whenever possible.		
3.	Provides privacy.		
4.	Adjusts bed to lowest position and locks bed wheels. Assists client to sitting position with feet flat on floor. Lets client sit for a few minutes. Puts nonskid shoes on client.		
5.	Stands in front of and faces client.		
6.	Places transfer belt around client's waist over clothing and grasps belt on both sides with hands in upward position.		
7.	If client needs help, braces client's lower extremities and bends knees. Has client lean forward and push down on bed with hands. Rocks weight onto back foot to assist client to standing position on count of 3.		
8.	Walks slightly behind and to one side of client, on weaker side, while holding on to transfer belt. Asks client to look forward, not down at feet.		
9.	Observes client's strength and provides chair if client becomes tired.		
10.	Returns client to bed or chair and removes transfer belt. Positions client comfortably. Leaves bed in lowest position.		
11.	Washes hands.		
12.	Documents procedure and any observations.		

Date Reviewed ______ Instructor Signature ______

Date Performed ______ Instructor Signature ______

Assisting with ambulation for a client using a cane, walker, or crutches

		yes	no
1.	Washes hands.		
2.	Explains procedure to client, speaking clearly, slowly, and directly. Maintains face-to-face contact whenever possible.		
3.	Provides privacy.		
4.	Adjusts bed to lowest position and locks bed wheels. Assists client to sitting position with feet flat on floor. Lets client sit for a few minutes. Puts nonskid shoes on client.		
5.	Stands in front of and faces client.		

Name: ______________________

6.	Places transfer belt around client's waist over clothing and grasps belt on both sides with hands in upward position.		
7.	Braces client's lower extremities and bends knees. Assists client to stand.		
8.	Helps as needed with ambulation with cane, walker, or crutches, walking slightly behind or on the client's weaker side.		
9.	Watches for obstacles in the client's path. Asks client to look forward, not down at feet.		
10.	Lets the client set the pace, encouraging rest as necessary.		
11.	Returns client to bed or chair and removes transfer belt. Positions client comfortably. Leaves bed in lowest position.		
12.	Washes hands.		
13.	Documents procedure and any observations.		

Date Reviewed ______ Instructor Signature ______

Date Performed ______ Instructor Signature ______

Giving a back massage

		yes	no
1.	Washes hands.		
2.	Explains procedure to client, speaking clearly, slowly, and directly. Maintains face-to-face contact whenever possible.		
3.	Provides privacy.		
4.	Adjusts bed to a safe working level. Lowers head of bed. Locks bed wheels.		
5.	Positions client to lie on side or stomach. Covers client with blanket and folds back bed covers, exposing client's back to the top of the buttocks.		
6.	Warms lotion and hands. Pours lotion onto hands and rubs hands together. Warns client that lotion may still feel cool.		
7.	Starting at the upper part of the buttocks, makes long, smooth upward strokes with both hands. Circles hands up along spine, shoulders, and then back down along the outer edges of the back. At buttocks, makes another circle up to the shoulders without taking hands off client's skin. Repeats for 3 to 5 minutes.		
8.	Starting at the base of the spine, makes kneading motions using the first two fingers and thumb of each hand. Circles hands up along spine, circling at shoulders and buttocks.		
9.	Gently massages bony areas. Massages around any red areas, rather than on them.		
10.	Lets client know when back rub is almost completed.		
11.	Dries the back.		
12.	Removes blanket or towel, assists client with getting dressed, and positions client comfortably. Returns bed to lowest position.		
13.	Stores lotion and puts dirty linens in hamper.		
14.	Washes hands.		
15.	Documents procedure and any observations.		

Date Reviewed ______ Instructor Signature ______

Date Performed ______ Instructor Signature ______

Name: ____________________

13
Personal Care Skills

Helping the client transfer to the bathtub		yes	no
1.	Washes hands.		
2.	Explains procedure to client, speaking clearly, slowly, and directly. Maintains face-to-face contact whenever possible.		
3.	Helps client to the bathroom.		
4.	Provides privacy.		
5.	Seats client in chair facing tub. If using wheelchair, locks brakes, and removes footrests.		
6.	Asks client to place legs one at a time over sides of tub.		
7.	Assists client to sitting position on edge of tub.		
8.	Lowers client into tub or onto tub chair, assisting as necessary.		
9.	Reverses procedure to help client out of tub.		
10.	Washes hands.		
11.	Documents procedure and any observations.		

Date Reviewed ____________ Instructor Signature ____________

Date Performed ____________ Instructor Signature ____________

Helping the ambulatory client take a shower or tub bath		yes	no
1.	Washes hands.		
2.	Explains procedure to client, speaking clearly, slowly, and directly. Maintains face-to-face contact whenever possible.		
3.	Cleans tub or shower if necessary, places mat, and sets up tub or shower chair. Places nonskid rug next to tub or shower.		
4.	Provides privacy.		
5.	Fills tub halfway with warm water (no higher than 105°F) or adjusts shower water temperature. Has client test water temperature and adjusts as necessary.		
6.	Puts on gloves.		
7.	Assists client to undress, as needed, and helps client transfer to tub or shower.		
8.	If client is able to bathe alone, places supplies and signal near client. Checks on client every 5 minutes. If client is weak, stays in bathroom.		
9.	If showering, stays with client and assists.		
10.	Assists client as necessary, washing from clean to dirty areas. Makes sure all soap is rinsed off.		
11.	Assists with shampooing as needed.		
12.	Helps client out and assists client with drying if necessary.		
13.	Helps client get dressed and, if the client is tired, back to bed.		
14.	Cleans tub. Places soiled laundry in laundry hamper.		
15.	Removes and discards gloves. Washes hands.		
16.	Stores supplies.		
17.	Documents procedure and any observations.		

Date Reviewed ____________ Instructor Signature ____________

Date Performed ____________ Instructor Signature ____________

Name: ____________________

Giving a complete bed bath

		yes	no
1.	Washes hands.		
2.	Explains procedure to client, speaking clearly, slowly, and directly. Maintains face-to-face contact whenever possible.		
3.	Provides privacy.		
4.	Makes sure room is a comfortable temperature. Adjusts bed to a safe working level. Locks bed wheels.		
5.	Asks client to remove eyeglasses and jewelry. Offers bedpan.		
6.	Places blanket over client and removes or folds back top bedding while keeping client covered. Removes top clothing while keeping client covered. Puts clothing in hamper.		
7.	Fills basin and checks temperature. Has client test water temperature and adjusts if necessary.		
8.	Puts on gloves.		
9.	Asks and assists client to participate in washing.		
10.	Uncovers only one part of the body at a time. Places a towel under the body part being washed.		
11.	Washes, rinses, and dries one part of the body at a time. Starts at the head, works down, and completes front first. Uses a clean area of the washcloth for each stroke.		
	Eyes, Face, Ears, and Neck: Washes face with wet washcloth (no soap). Begins with eye farther away, and washes inner to outer area, using a different area of the washcloth for each stroke. Washes the face from the middle outward using firm but gentle strokes. Washes ears and behind the ears and washes neck. Rinses and pats dry.		
	Arms and Axillae: Begins with arm farther away, and washes upper arm and underarm. Uses long strokes from the shoulder down to the wrist. Rinses and pats dry. Repeats for other arm.		
	Hands: Washes the far hand in a basin. Cleans under nails. Rinses and pats dry, including between the fingers. Gives nail care. Repeats for other hand. Applies lotion.		
	Chest: Places towel across the chest. Lifts the towel only enough to wash the chest, rinse it, and pat dry. For a female client: washes, rinses, and dries breasts and under breasts.		
	Abdomen: Keeps towel across the chest and folds blanket down so that it still covers genital area. Washes abdomen, rinses, and pats dry. Covers with a towel and pulls the blanket up to the chin and removes the towel.		

Name: ____________________

	Legs and Feet: Exposes the far leg and places towel under it. Washes the thigh, using long, downward strokes. Rinses and pats dry. Does the same from the knee to the ankle. Places another towel under the far foot and washes foot and between the toes in a basin. Rinses foot and pats dry, making sure area between toes is dry. Gives nail care if it has been assigned. Applies lotion if ordered but not between the toes. Repeats for other leg and foot.		
	Back: Helps client move to the center of the bed, and raises the far side rail. Then turns client onto his side, toward the raised side rail. Returns to working side so client's back is facing self. Washes neck and back with long, downward strokes. Rinses and pats dry. Applies lotion if ordered.		
12.	Places towel under buttocks and upper thighs. Helps client turn onto back. Removes and discards gloves. Washes hands and puts on clean gloves before washing perineal area.		
13.	***Perineal area and buttocks:*** Changes bath water. Washes, rinses, and dries perineal area, working from front to back.		
	For a female client: Washes the perineum with small amount of soap and water from front to back, using single strokes. Uses a clean area of washcloth or clean washcloth for each stroke. Working from front to back, wipes one side of the labia majora. Then wipes the other side, using a clean part of the cloth. Gently separates the labia majora and wipes from front to back on one side. Then wipes from front to back on the other side. Wipes from front to back down the center. Cleans the perineum last with a front to back motion. Rinses the area thoroughly in the same way, making sure all soap is removed. Dries entire perineal area moving from front to back, using a blotting motion with the towel. Asks client to turn on her side. Washes, rinses, and dries buttocks and anal area. Cleans anal area without contaminating the perineal area.		
	For a male client: If client is uncircumcised, pulls back the foreskin first. Gently pushes skin toward the base of penis. Holds the penis by the shaft and washes in a circular motion from the tip down to the base. Uses a clean area of washcloth or clean washcloth for each stroke. Rinses the penis and pats dry. If client is uncircumcised, gently returns foreskin to normal position. Then washes the scrotum and groin. Rinses and pats dry. Asks client to turn on his side. Washes, rinses, and dries buttocks and anal area. Cleans anal area without contaminating the perineal area.		

14.	Covers client. Places soiled washcloths and towels in proper container. Empties, rinses, and dries basin.		
15.	Removes and discards gloves. Washes hands.		
16.	Gives back rub if time permits.		
17.	Assists client with grooming as necessary. Returns bed to lowest position.		
18.	Stores everything. Places signaling device within reach. Dons clean gloves if sheets need to be changed.		
19.	Washes hands.		
20.	Documents procedure and any observations.		

Date Reviewed ____________ Instructor Signature ____________

Date Performed ____________ Instructor Signature ____________

Shampooing hair

		yes	no
1.	Washes hands.		
2.	Explains procedure to client, speaking clearly, slowly, and directly. Maintains face-to-face contact whenever possible.		
3.	Provides privacy. Makes sure that room is a comfortable temperature.		
4.	Tests water temperature and has client check water temperature. Adjusts if necessary.		
5.	Positions client in sink, tub, shower, or bed, and wets hair.		
6.	Applies shampoo, and massages scalp with fingertips (not fingernails).		
7.	Rinses hair thoroughly. Applies and rinses conditioner as needed.		
8.	Wraps client's hair in towel. Dries client's face and neck.		
9.	Removes towel and gently rubs scalp and hair. Combs or brushes hair.		
10.	Dries and styles hair.		
11.	Washes and stores equipment. Places soiled washcloths and towels in proper container.		
12.	Washes hands.		
13.	Documents procedure and any observations.		

Date Reviewed ____________ Instructor Signature ____________

Date Performed ____________ Instructor Signature ____________

Providing fingernail care

		yes	no
1.	Washes hands.		
2.	Explains procedure to client, speaking clearly, slowly, and directly. Maintains face-to-face contact whenever possible.		
3.	Provides privacy.		
4.	Adjusts bed to a safe working level. Locks bed wheels.		
5.	Removes rings and nail polish if necessary.		
6.	Fills basin and checks temperature. Has client test water temperature and adjusts if necessary.		
7.	Puts on gloves.		
8.	Soaks hands and nails for at least 5 minutes.		
9.	Removes hands from water. Washes hands with soapy washcloth. Rinses. Dries client's hands with a towel, including between fingers. Removes basin.		
10.	Cleans under nails with orangewood stick. Wipes orangewood stick on towel after each nail. Washes the hands again and dries, including between fingers.		

Name: ___________________________

11.	Shapes fingernails with an emery board or nail file moving in one direction only. Finishes with nails smooth and free of rough edges. Applies lotion. Removes excess lotion and replaces rings on fingers.		
12.	Discards water and rinses and dries basin. Places towels in proper place and stores supplies. Returns bed to lowest position.		
13.	Removes and discards gloves. Washes hands.		
14.	Documents procedure and any observations.		

Date Reviewed ________ Instructor Signature ________

Date Performed ________ Instructor Signature ________

Providing foot care

		yes	no
1.	Washes hands.		
2.	Explains procedure to client, speaking clearly, slowly, and directly. Maintains face-to-face contact whenever possible.		
3.	Provides privacy.		
4.	Adjusts bed to a safe working level. Locks bed wheels.		
5.	Fills basin and checks temperature. Has client test water temperature and adjusts if necessary.		
6.	Places basin on a bath mat or bath towel on the floor or on a towel at the foot of the bed. Supports foot and ankle throughout the procedure.		
7.	Puts on gloves.		
8.	Removes client's socks. Submerges client's feet in the water.		
9.	Removes one foot from water. Washes entire foot, including between the toes and around nail beds with soapy washcloth.		
10.	Rinses and dries entire foot, including between the toes.		
11.	Repeats steps for other foot.		
12.	Applies lotion to the feet (except between toes).		
13.	Helps client put on socks.		
14.	Discards water and rinses and dries basin. Places towels in proper place and stores supplies. Returns bed to lowest position.		
15.	Removes and discards gloves. Washes hands.		
16.	Documents procedure and any observations.		

Date Reviewed ________ Instructor Signature ________

Date Performed ________ Instructor Signature ________

Shaving a client

		yes	no
1.	Washes hands.		
2.	Explains procedure to client, speaking clearly, slowly, and directly. Maintains face-to-face contact whenever possible.		
3.	Provides privacy.		
4.	Places equipment within reach. Places client in an upright position. Adjusts bed to a safe working level. Locks bed wheels. Places towel across client's chest.		
5.	Puts on gloves.		

6.	***If using a safety or disposable razor,*** softens beard, lathers face, holds skin taut, and shaves in direction of hair growth. Rinses blade often. Rinses and dries face. Offers mirror.		
	If using an electric razor, turns it on, holds skin taut, and shaves with smooth, even movements. Shaves back and forth in direction of beard growth with foil shaver. Shaves in circular motion with three-head shaver. Shaves the chin and under the chin. Offers mirror.		
7.	Applies aftershave lotion if client wants it.		
8.	Puts towel and linens in hamper. Returns bed to lowest position. Cleans and stores equipment properly.		
9.	Removes and discards gloves. Washes hands.		
10.	Makes sure the area and the client's skin and clothing are free of loose hairs.		
11.	Documents procedure and any observations.		

Date Reviewed ____________ Instructor Signature ____________

Date Performed ____________ Instructor Signature ____________

Dressing a client

		yes	no
1.	Washes hands.		
2.	Explains procedure to client, speaking clearly, slowly, and directly. Maintains face-to-face contact whenever possible.		
3.	Provides privacy.		
4.	If client is in bed, raises head of bed to get client into an upright sitting position. Adjusts bed to a safe working level. Locks bed wheels.		
5.	Places blanket over client and folds back bedding to the foot of bed. Removes gown or top, keeping client covered. Takes clothes off stronger side first, then weaker side. Places gown in hamper. Moves blanket down to cover the lower body.		
6.	Helps put weaker arm through sleeve of top of client's choosing, then puts stronger arm through. Smooths top down and fastens it.		
7.	Removes blanket and places it in hamper. Helps put on skirt or pants of client's choosing, putting weaker leg through first, then stronger leg. Fastens pants or skirt.		
8.	Puts sock on weaker foot, then on stronger foot. Makes sure there are no wrinkles or twists.		
9.	Places bed in lowest position and has client sit on the side of the bed with legs dangling. Starting with weaker foot, puts on nonskid shoe and fastens it. Puts on second shoe and fastens it.		
10.	Finishes with client dressed appropriately, with zippers and buttons fastened. Leaves bed in lowest position.		
11.	Washes hands.		
12.	Documents procedure and any observations.		

Date Reviewed ____________ Instructor Signature ____________

Date Performed ____________ Instructor Signature ____________

Name: ____________________

Providing oral care		yes	no
1.	Washes hands.		
2.	Explains procedure to client, speaking clearly, slowly, and directly. Maintains face-to-face contact whenever possible.		
3.	Provides privacy.		
4.	If in bed, raises head of bed to get client into an upright sitting position. Adjusts bed to a safe working level. Locks bed wheels.		
5.	Puts on gloves. Places towel across chest.		
6.	Removes dental bridgework.		
7.	Wets brush and puts a small amount of toothpaste on brush.		
8.	Gently brushes teeth, including tongue and all surfaces of teeth and gumline. First brushes inner, outer, and chewing surfaces of the upper teeth, then does the same with the lower teeth. Brushes tongue.		
9.	Gives client water to rinse her mouth and has client spit water into emesis basin.		
10.	Wipes client's mouth and removes towel.		
11.	Replaces dental bridgework. Applies moisturizer to lips.		
12.	Rinses toothbrush and places in proper container. Discards water, and rinses and dries basin. Places towels in hamper and stores supplies. Returns bed to lowest position.		
13.	Removes and discards gloves. Washes hands.		
14.	Documents procedure and any observations.		

Date Reviewed ____________ Instructor Signature ____________

Date Performed ____________ Instructor Signature ____________

Providing oral care for the unconscious client		yes	no
1.	Washes hands.		
2.	Explains procedure to client, speaking clearly, slowly, and directly. Maintains face-to-face contact whenever possible.		
3.	Provides privacy.		
4.	Adjusts bed to a safe working level. Locks bed wheels.		
5.	Puts on gloves.		
6.	Turns client on his side and places a towel under cheek and chin. Places basin next to cheek and chin.		
7.	Holds mouth open with tongue depressor. Dips swab in solution and squeezes swab to remove excess solution. Wipes inner, outer, and chewing surfaces of upper and lower teeth, gums, tongue, and inside surfaces of mouth. Changes swab often. Repeats until clean.		
8.	Rinses with clean swab dipped in water. Squeezes swab first to remove excess water.		
9.	Removes towel and basin. Pats face dry. Applies moisturizer to lips.		
10.	Discards water, and rinses and dries basin. Places towels in hamper and stores supplies. Returns bed to lowest position.		
11.	Removes and discards gloves. Washes hands.		

12.	Documents procedure and any observations.		

Date Reviewed ______ Instructor Signature ______

Date Performed ______ Instructor Signature ______

Flossing teeth

		yes	no
1.	Washes hands.		
2.	Explains procedure to client, speaking clearly, slowly, and directly. Maintains face-to-face contact whenever possible.		
3.	Provides privacy.		
4.	If in bed, raises head of bed to get client into an upright sitting position. Adjusts bed to a safe working level. Locks bed wheels.		
5.	Puts on gloves.		
6.	Wraps floss around index fingers.		
7.	Flosses teeth, starting with the back teeth.		
8.	Uses clean area of floss after every two teeth.		
9.	Offers water periodically and offers a towel when done.		
10.	Discards floss, discards water, and rinses and dries basin. Places towels in hamper and stores supplies. Returns bed to lowest position.		
11.	Removes and discards gloves. Washes hands.		
12.	Documents procedure and any observations.		

Date Reviewed ______ Instructor Signature ______

Date Performed ______ Instructor Signature ______

Cleaning and storing dentures

		yes	no
1.	Washes hands.		
2.	Explains procedure to client, speaking clearly, slowly, and directly. Maintains face-to-face contact whenever possible.		
3.	Provides privacy.		
4.	Puts on gloves.		
5.	Lines sink or basin with towel and partially fills with water.		
6.	Removes lower denture properly if client is unable and places it in denture cup filled with moderate/cool water.		
7.	Removes upper denture properly and places it in denture cup filled with moderate/cool water.		
8.	Rinses dentures in clean, moderate/cool running water. Applies denture cleanser to toothbrush and brushes all surfaces. Rinses all surfaces under clean, moderate/cool running water.		
9.	Rinses denture cup and lid.		
10.	If client prefers, soaks dentures in solution.		
11.	Stores dentures in moderate/cool water or solution in labeled denture cup, or returns dentures to client.		
12.	Rinses toothbrush and places in proper container. Washes and stores supplies.		
13.	Removes and discards gloves. Washes hands.		
14.	Documents procedure and any observations.		

Date Reviewed ______ Instructor Signature ______

Date Performed ______ Instructor Signature ______

Name: ______________________

Reinserting dentures

		yes	no
1.	Washes hands.		
2.	Explains procedure to client, speaking clearly, slowly, and directly. Maintains face-to-face contact whenever possible.		
3.	Provides privacy.		
4.	Positions client in upright position.		
5.	Puts on gloves.		
6.	Applies denture cream to dentures.		
7.	Inserts upper denture at an angle, pressing it firmly onto upper gumline.		
8.	Inserts lower denture, pressing it firmly onto the lower gumline.		
9.	Offers client face towel.		
10.	Rinses and stores denture cup. Places towel in hamper and stores supplies.		
11.	Removes and discards gloves. Washes hands.		
12.	Documents procedure and any observations.		

Date Reviewed ______ Instructor Signature ______

Date Performed ______ Instructor Signature ______

Assisting a client with use of a bedpan

		yes	no
1.	Washes hands.		
2.	Explains procedure to client, speaking clearly, slowly, and directly. Maintains face-to-face contact whenever possible.		
3.	Provides privacy.		
4.	Adjusts bed to a safe working level. Raises far side rail (if available). Lowers head of bed. Locks bed wheels.		
5.	Puts on gloves.		
6.	Covers client with cotton blanket and places a bed protector under client's buttocks and hips.		
7.	Asks client to remove undergarments or helps client to do so.		
8.	Places bedpan near hips. Positions standard bedpan with wider end aligned with the buttocks. Positions fracture pan with handle toward foot of bed. Slides bedpan under hips.		
9.	Removes and discards gloves. Washes hands. Raises head of bed after placing bedpan. Leaves side rails up and returns bed to lowest position.		
10.	Provides client with supplies. Asks client to clean his hands after bedpan use. Leaves room and closes door until client calls.		
11.	When called, returns and washes hands. Puts on clean gloves. Raises bed to a safe working level and lowers head of bed. Removes and covers bedpan. If client is unable, gives perineal care.		
12.	Helps client put on undergarments. Covers client and removes cotton blanket. Discards soiled supplies. Places linens in hamper.		
13.	Takes bedpan to the bathroom. Notes contents before flushing. Empties bedpan into toilet. Rinses bedpan with cold water and empties. Flushes toilet. Cleans bedpan with hot, soapy water and stores.		
14.	Removes and discards gloves. Washes hands.		
15.	Returns bed to lowest position.		

Name: ______________________

16.	Documents procedure and any observations.		

Date Reviewed ______ Instructor Signature ______

Date Performed ______ Instructor Signature ______

Assisting a client with a urinal

		yes	no
1.	Washes hands.		
2.	Explains procedure to client, speaking clearly, slowly, and directly. Maintains face-to-face contact whenever possible.		
3.	Provides privacy.		
4.	Adjusts the bed to a safe working level. Locks bed wheels.		
5.	Puts on gloves.		
6.	Places bed protector under client's buttocks and hips.		
7.	Hands urinal to client or places it if client is unable. Replaces covers.		
8.	Removes and discards gloves. Washes hands. Raises head of bed after placing urinal. Leaves side rails up and returns bed to lowest position.		
9.	Gives client a bell and wipes. Asks client to clean his hands after urinal use. Leaves room and closes door until client calls.		
10.	When called, returns and washes hands. Puts on clean gloves. Raises bed to a safe working level. Removes and discards supplies.		
11.	Takes urinal to the bathroom. Notes contents before flushing. Rinses urinal, flushes toilet, and stores urinal.		
12.	Removes and discards gloves. Washes hands.		
13.	Returns bed to lowest position.		
14.	Documents procedure and any observations.		

Date Reviewed ______ Instructor Signature ______

Date Performed ______ Instructor Signature ______

Helping a client use a portable commode or toilet

		yes	no
1.	Washes hands.		
2.	Explains procedure to client, speaking clearly, slowly, and directly. Maintains face-to-face contact whenever possible.		
3.	Provides privacy.		
4.	Locks commode wheels. Adjusts the bed to lowest position. Locks bed wheels. Makes sure client is wearing nonskid shoes and helps client to bathroom or commode, using transfer belt as needed.		
5.	Puts on gloves.		
6.	Helps client remove clothing and sit down. Provides client with supplies and asks client to clean his hands. Removes and discards gloves. Washes hands. Leaves room and closes door until client calls.		
7.	When called, returns and washes hands. Puts on clean gloves. Gives perineal care if help is needed. Discards soiled items.		
8.	Removes and discards gloves. Washes hands.		
9.	Helps client back to bed and puts on clean gloves.		
10.	Removes waste container and notes contents. Empties into toilet and flushes.		

Name: ________________________

11.	Cleans container, rinsing first with cold water, then hot, soapy water.		
12.	Removes and discards gloves. Washes hands.		
13.	Documents procedure and any observations.		

_______ Date Reviewed _______ Instructor Signature

_______ Date Performed _______ Instructor Signature

14 Core Healthcare Skills

Measuring and recording an oral temperature			
		yes	no
1.	Washes hands.		
2.	Explains procedure to client, speaking clearly, slowly, and directly. Maintains face-to-face contact whenever possible.		
3.	Provides privacy.		
4.	Puts on gloves.		
5.	***Digital thermometer:*** Puts on disposable sheath. Turns on thermometer and waits until ready sign appears. ***Electronic thermometer:*** Removes probe from base unit and puts on probe cover. ***Mercury-free thermometer:*** Holds thermometer by stem. Shakes thermometer down to below the lowest number.		
6.	***Digital thermometer:*** Inserts end of thermometer into client's mouth, under tongue and to one side. ***Electronic thermometer:*** Inserts end of thermometer into client's mouth, under tongue and to one side. ***Mercury-free thermometer:*** Puts on disposable sheath if available. Inserts bulb end of thermometer into client's mouth, under tongue and to one side.		
7.	***For all thermometers:*** Asks client to hold thermometer in his mouth with his lips closed. ***Digital thermometer:*** Holds in place until thermometer blinks or beeps. ***Electronic thermometer:*** Holds in place until tone or light signals temperature has been read. ***Mercury-free thermometer:*** Holds in place for at least 3 minutes.		
8.	***Digital thermometer:*** Removes thermometer. Reads temperature on display screen and remembers reading. ***Electronic thermometer:*** Reads temperature on display screen and remembers reading. Removes probe. ***Mercury-free thermometer:*** Removes thermometer. Wipes with tissue from stem to bulb or removes sheath. Discards tissue or sheath. Reads temperature and remembers reading.		

Name: ______________________________

9.	***Digital thermometer:*** Using a tissue, removes and discards sheath. Stores thermometer. ***Electronic thermometer:*** Presses the eject button to discard the cover. Returns probe to holder. ***Mercury-free thermometer:*** Cleans thermometer according to policy. Rinses, dries, and stores thermometer.		
10.	Removes and discards gloves. Washes hands.		
11.	Documents temperature, date, time, and method used (oral).		

Date Reviewed ______ Instructor Signature ______

Date Performed ______ Instructor Signature ______

Measuring and recording a rectal temperature			
		yes	no
1.	Washes hands.		
2.	Explains procedure to client, speaking clearly, slowly, and directly. Maintains face-to-face contact whenever possible.		
3.	Provides privacy.		
4.	Adjusts bed to a safe working level. Locks bed wheels. Assists client to left-lying position.		
5.	Folds back linens to only expose rectal area.		
6.	Puts on gloves.		
7.	***Digital thermometer:*** Puts on disposable sheath. Turns on thermometer and waits until ready sign appears. ***Electronic thermometer:*** Removes probe from base unit and puts on probe cover. ***Mercury-free thermometer:*** Holds thermometer by stem. Shakes thermometer down to below the lowest number. Puts on disposable sheath.		
8.	Applies a small amount of lubricant to tip of bulb or probe cover.		
9.	Separates buttocks. Gently inserts thermometer into rectum 1/2 to 1 inch. Replaces sheet over buttocks. Holds on to thermometer at all times while taking temperature.		
10.	***Digital thermometer:*** Holds thermometer in place until thermometer blinks or beeps. ***Electronic thermometer:*** Holds in place until tone or light signals temperature has been read. ***Mercury-free thermometer:*** Holds thermometer in place for at least 3 minutes.		
11.	Removes thermometer and wipes thermometer with tissue from stem to bulb or removes sheath. Discards tissue or sheath.		
12.	Reads temperature and remembers reading.		

Name: ______________________

13.	***Digital thermometer:*** Cleans and stores thermometer. ***Electronic thermometer:*** Presses the eject button to discard the cover. Cleans probe and returns it to holder. ***Mercury-free thermometer:*** Cleans thermometer according to policy. Rinses, dries, and stores thermometer.		
14.	Removes and discards gloves. Washes hands. Returns bed to lowest position.		
15.	Washes hands.		
16.	Documents temperature, date, time, and method used (rectal).		

Date Reviewed ______ Instructor Signature ______

Date Performed ______ Instructor Signature ______

Measuring and recording a tympanic temperature

		yes	no
1.	Washes hands.		
2.	Explains procedure to client, speaking clearly, slowly, and directly. Maintains face-to-face contact whenever possible.		
3.	Provides privacy.		
4.	Puts on gloves.		
5.	Places disposable probe cover over earpiece of thermometer.		
6.	Positions client's head properly and gently pulls up and back on the outside edge of the ear. Inserts covered probe and presses the button.		
7.	Holds thermometer in place until it blinks or beeps.		
8.	Reads temperature and remembers reading.		
9.	Discards sheath and stores thermometer properly.		
10.	Removes and discards gloves. Washes hands.		
11.	Documents temperature, date, time, and method used (tympanic).		

Date Reviewed ______ Instructor Signature ______

Date Performed ______ Instructor Signature ______

Measuring and recording an axillary temperature

		yes	no
1.	Washes hands.		
2.	Explains procedure to client, speaking clearly, slowly, and directly. Maintains face-to-face contact whenever possible.		
3.	Provides privacy.		
4.	Adjusts bed to a safe working level. Locks bed wheels.		
5.	Puts on gloves.		
6.	Removes client's arm from clothing and wipes axillary area with tissues.		
7.	***Digital thermometer:*** Puts on disposable sheath. Turns on thermometer and waits until ready sign appears. ***Electronic thermometer:*** Removes probe from base unit and puts on probe cover. ***Mercury-free thermometer:*** Holds thermometer by stem. Shakes thermometer down to below the lowest number. Puts on disposable sheath.		

Name: ______________________

8.	Positions thermometer in center of armpit and folds client's arm over chest.		
9.	***Digital thermometer:*** Holds in place until thermometer blinks or beeps. ***Electronic thermometer:*** Holds in place until tone or light signals temperature has been read. ***Mercury-free thermometer:*** Holds in place for 8 to 10 minutes.		
10.	***Digital thermometer:*** Removes thermometer. Reads temperature on display screen and remembers reading. ***Electronic thermometer:*** Reads temperature on display screen and remembers reading. Removes probe. ***Mercury-free thermometer:*** Removes thermometer. Wipes with tissue from stem to bulb or removes sheath. Discards tissue or sheath. Reads temperature and remembers reading.		
11.	***Digital thermometer:*** Removes and disposes of sheath with a tissue. Stores thermometer. ***Electronic thermometer:*** Presses the eject button to discard the cover. Cleans probe and returns it to holder. ***Mercury-free thermometer:*** Cleans thermometer according to policy. Rinses, dries, and stores thermometer.		
12.	Returns bed to lowest position.		
13.	Removes and discards gloves. Washes hands.		
14.	Documents temperature, date, time, and method used (axillary).		

Date Reviewed ______ Instructor Signature ______

Date Performed ______ Instructor Signature ______

Measuring and recording a temporal artery temperature

		yes	no
1.	Washes hands.		
2.	Explains procedure to client, speaking clearly, slowly, and directly. Maintains face-to-face contact whenever possible.		
3.	Provides privacy.		
4.	Turns on thermometer. Places it flat on client's forehead, usually midway between eyebrow and hairline.		
5.	Presses and holds scan button. Gently sweeps thermometer across client's forehead, maintaining contact with skin. Releases scan button.		
6.	Reads and remembers temperature on display screen.		
7.	Wipes thermometer clean using alcohol swab or cotton-tipped applicator moistened in alcohol.		
8.	Washes hands.		
9.	Documents temperature, date, time, and method used (temporal artery).		

Date Reviewed ______ Instructor Signature ______

Date Performed ______ Instructor Signature ______

Name: ______________________

Counting and recording apical pulse			
		yes	no
1.	Washes hands.		
2.	Explains procedure to client, speaking clearly, slowly, and directly. Maintains face-to-face contact whenever possible.		
3.	Provides privacy.		
4.	Wipes diaphragm and earpieces of stethoscope with alcohol wipes. Fits earpieces of stethoscope snugly in ears and places flat metal diaphragm on left side of chest, just below the nipple.		
5.	Counts heartbeats for 1 full minute.		
6.	Counts client's respirations with stethoscope still in place.		
7.	Washes hands.		
8.	Documents pulse rate, date, time, and method used (apical). Documents respiratory rate and the character of breathing.		
9.	Cleans and stores stethoscope.		
10.	Washes hands.		

Date Reviewed ______ Instructor Signature ______

Date Performed ______ Instructor Signature ______

Counting and recording radial pulse and counting and recording respirations			
		yes	no
1.	Washes hands.		
2.	Explains procedure to client, speaking clearly, slowly, and directly. Maintains face-to-face contact whenever possible.		
3.	Provides privacy.		
4.	Places fingertips of index finger and middle finger on the thumb side of client's wrist to locate radial pulse.		
5.	Counts beats for 1 full minute.		
6.	Keeping fingertips on client's wrist, counts respirations for 1 full minute.		
7.	Washes hands.		
8.	Documents pulse rate, date, time, and method used (radial). Documents respiratory rate and the character of breathing.		

Date Reviewed ______ Instructor Signature ______

Date Performed ______ Instructor Signature ______

Measuring and recording blood pressure manually			
		yes	no
1.	Washes hands.		
2.	Explains procedure to client, speaking clearly, slowly, and directly. Maintains face-to-face contact whenever possible.		
3.	Provides privacy.		
4.	Wipes diaphragm and earpieces of stethoscope with alcohol wipes.		
5.	Asks client to roll up sleeve. Positions client's arm with palm up. The arm should be level with the heart.		
6.	With the valve open, squeezes the cuff to make sure it is completely deflated.		
7.	Places blood pressure cuff snugly on client's upper arm, with the center of the cuff placed over the brachial artery.		

8.	Asks client to remain still and quiet during measurement. Locates the brachial pulse with fingertips.		
9.	Places earpieces of stethoscope in ears and places diaphragm of stethoscope over brachial artery.		
10.	Closes the valve (clockwise) until it stops. Inflates cuff to between 160 mm Hg and 180 mm Hg. If a beat is heard immediately upon cuff deflation, completely deflates cuff. Reinflates cuff to no more than 200 mm Hg.		
11.	Opens the valve slightly with thumb and index finger. Deflates cuff slowly.		
12.	Watches gauge and listens for sound of pulse.		
13.	Remembers the reading at which the first clear pulse sound is heard. This is the systolic pressure.		
14.	Continues listening for a change or muffling of pulse sound. The point of a change or the point the sound disappears is the diastolic pressure. Remembers this reading.		
15.	Opens the valve to deflate cuff completely. Removes cuff.		
16.	Washes hands.		
17.	Documents both systolic and diastolic pressures. Notes which arm was used.		
18.	Cleans stethoscope. Stores equipment.		
19.	Washes hands.		

Date Reviewed ______ Instructor Signature ______

Date Performed ______ Instructor Signature ______

Measuring and recording blood pressure electronically

		yes	no
1.	Washes hands.		
2.	Explains procedure to client, speaking clearly, slowly, and directly. Maintains face-to-face contact whenever possible.		
3.	Provides privacy.		
4.	Asks client to roll up sleeve. Positions client's arm with palm up. The arm should be level with the heart.		
5.	Makes sure cuff is completely deflated. Places blood pressure cuff snugly on client's upper arm, with the center of the cuff placed over the brachial artery.		
6.	Asks client to remain still and quiet during measurement.		
7.	Turns on machine and presses start.		
8.	After measurement is complete, removes cuff.		
9.	Washes hands.		
10.	Documents both systolic and diastolic pressures. Notes which arm was used.		
11.	Stores equipment.		
12.	Washes hands.		

Date Reviewed ______ Instructor Signature ______

Date Performed ______ Instructor Signature ______

Measuring and recording weight of an ambulatory client

		yes	no
1.	Washes hands.		
2.	Explains procedure to client, speaking clearly, slowly, and directly. Maintains face-to-face contact whenever possible.		

Name: ______________________

3.	Provides privacy.		
4.	Sets scale on hard floor surface. Makes sure client is wearing nonskid shoes.		
5.	Starts with scale at 0.		
6.	Helps client to step on scale as necessary. Makes sure client is not holding, touching, or leaning against anything.		
7.	Determines client's weight. If using a bathroom scale, reads weight on display screen or when dial has stopped moving. If using a standing scale, balances the bar and adds numbers together.		
8.	Helps client to step off the scale and back to a comfortable position.		
9.	Washes hands.		
10.	Documents the weight in pounds (lb) or kilograms (kg).		
11.	Stores the scale.		
12.	Washes hands.		

Date Reviewed ______ Instructor Signature ______

Date Performed ______ Instructor Signature ______

Measuring and recording height of a client

		yes	no
1.	Washes hands.		
2.	Explains procedure to client, speaking clearly, slowly, and directly. Maintains face-to-face contact whenever possible.		
3.	Provides privacy.		
4.	Positions client straight in bed, flat on her back, with arms and legs at sides. Makes sure bedsheet is smooth underneath client.		
5.	Makes a small pencil mark at the top of client's head and at client's heel.		
6.	Measures distance between the two marks with a tape measure.		
7.	Washes hands.		
8.	Documents client's height.		
9.	Stores equipment.		
10.	Washes hands.		
	For clients who can get out of bed:		
1.	Washes hands.		
2.	Explains procedure to client, speaking clearly, slowly, and directly. Maintains face-to-face contact whenever possible.		
3.	Provides privacy.		
4.	Asks client to remove shoes and stand with his back against a wall and arms at his sides.		
5.	Makes a small pencil mark on the wall even with the top of the client's head.		
6.	Asks client to step away. Measures the distance between the pencil mark and the floor.		
7.	Washes hands.		
8.	Documents height.		
9.	Stores equipment.		
10.	Washes hands.		
	If using a standing scale:		
1.	Washes hands.		
2.	Explains procedure to client, speaking clearly, slowly, and directly. Maintains face-to-face contact whenever possible.		
3.	Provides privacy.		
4.	Makes sure client has on nonskid shoes and helps client to step onto scale, facing away from the scale.		

5.	With client standing straight, pulls up measuring rod and lowers it until it rests flat on client's head.		
6.	Determines client's height. Assists client to step off the scale and back to a comfortable position.		
7.	Washes hands.		
8.	Documents the height.		

Date Reviewed ____ Instructor Signature ____

Date Performed ____ Instructor Signature ____

Collecting a sputum specimen

		yes	no
1.	Washes hands.		
2.	Explains procedure to client, speaking clearly, slowly, and directly. Maintains face-to-face contact whenever possible.		
3.	Provides privacy.		
4.	Ensures client is standing or sitting upright. Puts on mask and gloves.		
5.	Stands behind or away from client. Gives client tissues to cover the mouth. Asks client to cough deeply and spit the sputum into the specimen container.		
6.	Covers container tightly, and wipes any sputum off the outside of the container. Discards tissues, applies label, places container in clean specimen bag, and seals bag.		
7.	Removes and discards gloves and mask.		
8.	Washes hands.		
9.	Documents procedure and any observations.		

Date Reviewed ____ Instructor Signature ____

Date Performed ____ Instructor Signature ____

Collecting a stool specimen

		yes	no
1.	Washes hands.		
2.	Explains procedure to client, speaking clearly, slowly, and directly. Maintains face-to-face contact whenever possible.		
3.	Provides privacy.		
4.	Puts on gloves.		
5.	Asks client not to urinate at the same time as moving bowels and not to put toilet paper in with the sample. Provides plastic bag to discard toilet paper separately.		
6.	Fits hat to toilet or commode or provides client with bedpan. Makes sure bed is in its lowest position. Provides client with supplies. Asks the client to call when he is finished.		
7.	Removes and discards gloves. Washes hands. Leaves the room and closes the door.		
8.	When called, returns and washes hands. Puts on clean gloves. Helps with perineal care if needed.		
9.	Uses tongue blades to take about 2 tablespoons of stool and puts stool in container without touching the inside. Covers container tightly, applies label, places in clean specimen bag, and seals the bag.		

Name: ______________

10.	Discards tongue blades. Empties and rinses bedpan or container and flushes toilet. Cleans and stores equipment.		
11.	Stores the specimen properly.		
12.	Removes and discards gloves. Washes hands.		
13.	Documents procedure and any observations.		

Date Reviewed ______ Instructor Signature ______

Date Performed ______ Instructor Signature ______

Collecting a routine urine specimen

		yes	no
1.	Washes hands.		
2.	Explains procedure to client, speaking clearly, slowly, and directly. Maintains face-to-face contact whenever possible.		
3.	Provides privacy.		
4.	Puts on gloves.		
5.	Fits hat to toilet or commode or provides client with bedpan or urinal. Asks client not to put toilet paper in with the sample. Provides plastic bag to discard toilet paper separately.		
6.	Makes sure bed is in its lowest position. Provides client with supplies. Asks the client to call when he is finished.		
7.	Removes and discards gloves. Washes hands. Leaves the room and closes the door.		
8.	When called, returns and washes hands. Puts on clean gloves. Helps with perineal care if needed.		
9.	Takes bedpan, urinal, or commode pail to the bathroom. Pours urine into specimen container, filling it at least halfway.		
10.	Covers container with lid. Wipe[illegible] off the outside with a paper towel and discards paper towel.		
11.	Applies label, places the container in a clean specimen bag, and seals bag.		
12.	Discards extra urine, rinses container, and flushes toilet. Cleans and stores equipment.		
13.	Removes and discards gloves. Washes hands.		
14.	Documents procedure and any observations.		

Date Reviewed ______ Instructor Signature ______

Date Performed ______ Instructor Signature ______

Collecting a clean-catch (midstream) urine specimen

		yes	no
1.	Washes hands.		
2.	Explains procedure to client, speaking clearly, slowly, and directly. Maintains face-to-face contact whenever possible.		
3.	Provides privacy.		
4.	Puts on gloves.		
5.	Opens specimen kit.		
6.	Cleans perineal area if help is needed.		
7.	Asks client to urinate into the bedpan, urinal, or toilet and to stop before urination is complete.		
8.	Places container under the urine stream and instructs client to start urinating again until container is at least half full. Has client finish urinating in bedpan, toilet, or urinal.		
9.	Gives perineal care if help is needed and asks client to clean hands.		

		yes	no
10.	Covers container with lid, wipes off outside with paper towel, and discards paper towel.		
11.	Applies label, places the container in a clean specimen bag, and seals bag.		
12.	Discards extra urine, rinses container, and flushes toilet. Cleans and stores equipment.		
13.	Removes and discards gloves. Washes hands.		
14.	Documents procedure and any observations.		

Date Reviewed ____________ Instructor Signature ____________

Date Performed ____________ Instructor Signature ____________

Collecting a 24-hour urine specimen

		yes	no
1.	Washes hands.		
2.	Explains procedure to client, speaking clearly, slowly, and directly. Maintains face-to-face contact whenever possible.		
3.	Provides privacy.		
4.	Asks client to completely empty the bladder. Discards urine and notes the exact time.		
5.	Washes hands and puts on gloves each time client voids.		
6.	Pours urine from bedpan, urinal, or hat into container, using the funnel as needed.		
7.	Assists client with perineal care and with washing hands after each voiding.		
8.	Asks client and family to save all urine and store properly after each voiding.		
9.	Cleans equipment after each voiding.		
10.	Removes and discards gloves. Washes hands.		
11.	Documents procedure and any observations.		

Date Reviewed ____________ Instructor Signature ____________

Date Performed ____________ Instructor Signature ____________

Measuring and recording intake and output

		yes	no
1.	***For measuring intake:*** Washes hands.		
2.	Explains procedure to client, speaking clearly, slowly, and directly. Maintains face-to-face contact whenever possible.		
3.	Provides privacy.		
4.	Measures amount of fluid client is served and notes on paper.		
5.	Measures leftover fluids and notes on paper.		
6.	Subtracts amount left over from amount served. Converts to milliliters (mL) as needed.		
7.	Documents amount of fluids consumed (in mL), time, and type of fluid in visit notes or I&O sheet.		
8.	Washes hands.		
1.	***For measuring output:*** Washes hands.		
2.	Puts on gloves.		
3.	Pours urine into measuring container. Measures amount of urine at eye level and notes amount on paper.		
4.	Discards urine. Rinses, cleans, and stores equipment.		
5.	Removes and discards gloves. Washes hands.		

Name: ______________________

6.	Documents the time and amount (in mL) of urine.		

Date Reviewed ________ Instructor Signature ________

Date Performed ________ Instructor Signature ________

Observing, reporting, and documenting emesis

		yes	no
1.	Puts on gloves.		
2.	Provides a basin and removes it when vomiting has stopped.		
3.	Removes soiled linens or clothes and replaces with fresh ones.		
4.	Measures and notes amount of vomitus if monitoring client's I&O.		
5.	Discards vomit in toilet unless vomit is red, has blood in it, or looks like wet coffee grounds. Washes and stores basin.		
6.	Removes and discards gloves. Washes hands.		
7.	Puts on clean gloves.		
8.	Provides comfort to client.		
9.	Launders soiled linens and clothes in hot water.		
10.	Removes and discards gloves.		
11.	Washes hands.		
12.	Documents time, amount, color, and consistency of vomitus.		
13.	Reports to supervisor immediately and gets instructions for diet.		

Date Reviewed ________ Instructor Signature ________

Date Performed ________ Instructor Signature ________

Providing urinary catheter care

		yes	no
1.	Washes hands.		
2.	Explains procedure to client, speaking clearly, slowly, and directly. Maintains face-to-face contact whenever possible.		
3.	Provides privacy.		
4.	Adjusts bed to a safe working level. Locks bed wheels. Lowers head of bed and positions client lying flat on back.		
5.	Removes or folds back top bedding, keeping client covered with bath blanket.		
6.	Checks water temperature. Has client test water temperature and adjusts if necessary.		
7.	Puts on gloves.		
8.	Places clean bed protector under client's perineal area, including her buttocks.		
9.	Exposes only the area necessary to clean the catheter.		
10.	Places towel under catheter tubing before washing.		
11.	Applies soap to washcloth and cleans area around meatus, using a clean area of the cloth for each stroke.		
12.	Holding catheter near meatus, cleans at least 4 inches of catheter. Moves in only one direction, away from meatus, and avoids tugging. Uses a clean area of the cloth for each stroke.		
13.	Dips clean washcloth in water and rinses area around meatus, using a clean area of washcloth for each stroke.		

14.	Dips clean washcloth in water and rinses at least 4 inches of catheter nearest meatus, moving away from meatus. Uses a clean area of washcloth for each stroke.		
15.	With a clean, dry towel, dries at least 4 inches of the catheter nearest the meatus, moving away from the meatus.		
16.	Removes bed protector and towel. Empties water into toilet and flushes. Places linen in proper containers. Cleans and stores basin.		
17.	Removes and discards gloves. Washes hands.		
18.	Removes bath blanket and replaces top covers. Returns bed to lowest position.		
19.	Helps client dress. Arranges covers. Checks that catheter tubing is free from kinks and twists and that it is securely taped to the leg.		
20.	Washes hands.		
21.	Documents procedure and any observations.		

Date Reviewed ________ Instructor Signature ________

Date Performed ________ Instructor Signature ________

Emptying the urinary catheter drainage bag

		yes	no
1.	Washes hands.		
2.	Explains procedure to client, speaking clearly, slowly, and directly. Maintains face-to-face contact whenever possible.		
3.	Provides privacy.		
4.	Puts on gloves.		
5.	Places measuring container on paper towel on floor under drainage bag.		
6.	Opens clamp on bag so urine flows into graduate.		
7.	Closes clamp and cleans drain spout. Replaces drain spout in its holder on the bag.		
8.	Goes into bathroom. Places graduate on a flat surface and measures at eye level. Notes amount and appearance of urine and empties it into toilet. Flushes toilet.		
9.	Cleans and stores graduate.		
10.	Removes and discards gloves. Washes hands.		
11.	Documents procedure and any observations.		

Date Reviewed ________ Instructor Signature ________

Date Performed ________ Instructor Signature ________

Changing a condom catheter

		yes	no
1.	Washes hands.		
2.	Explains procedure to client, speaking clearly, slowly, and directly. Maintains face-to-face contact whenever possible.		
3.	Provides privacy.		
4.	Adjusts bed to a safe working level. Locks bed wheels. Lowers head of bed and positions client lying flat on his back.		
5.	Removes or folds back bedding, keeping client covered with bath blanket.		
6.	Puts on gloves.		

Name: ____________________

		yes	no
7.	Places a clean bed protector under client's perineal area, including buttocks. Adjusts bath blanket to only expose genital area.		
8.	Removes condom catheter if one is in place, putting condom and tape in plastic bag.		
9.	Assists as necessary with perineal care.		
10.	Moves pubic hair away from penis. Places condom on penis and rolls toward base of penis, leaving space between drainage tip and glans of penis to prevent irritation.		
11.	Secures condom to penis with special tape applied in spiral manner.		
12.	Connects catheter tip to drainage tubing. Makes sure tubing is not twisted or kinked. Checks to see if bag is secured to the leg and makes sure drain is closed.		
13.	Removes and discards bed protector. Discards used supplies in plastic bag. Places soiled linen in proper container. Cleans and stores supplies.		
14.	Removes and discards gloves. Washes hands.		
15.	Removes bath blanket and replaces top covers. Returns bed to its lowest position. Washes hands.		
16.	Documents procedure and any observations.		

Date Reviewed ____________ Instructor Signature ____________

Date Performed ____________ Instructor Signature ____________

Applying a warm or cold compress

		yes	no
1.	Washes hands.		
2.	Explains procedure to client, speaking clearly, slowly, and directly. Maintains face-to-face contact whenever possible.		
3.	Provides privacy.		
4.	Fills the basin halfway with warm or cold water. For a warm compress, tests water temperature and has client check water temperature. Adjusts if necessary. Follows manufacturer instructions for commercial compress.		
5.	Places bed protector under area to be treated. Soaks washcloth, wrings it out, and applies to area needing compress. Covers warm compress with plastic wrap and towel. For cold compress, changes washcloths often.		
6.	Notes the time. Checks area every 5 minutes. Changes compress as needed.		
7.	Removes compress after 20 minutes, or if area is discolored, numb, or blistered, or if the client complains of pain or discomfort.		
8.	Discards disposable supplies and empties basin in toilet. Rinses, cleans, and stores basin and other supplies. Puts laundry in hamper.		
9.	Washes hands.		
10.	Documents time, length, and site of procedure and any observations.		

Date Reviewed ____________ Instructor Signature ____________

Date Performed ____________ Instructor Signature ____________

Name: ______________________

Administering a warm soak

		yes	no
1.	Washes hands.		
2.	Explains procedure to client, speaking clearly, slowly, and directly. Maintains face-to-face contact whenever possible.		
3.	Provides privacy.		
4.	Fills the basin halfway with warm water. Tests water temperature and has client check water temperature. Adjusts if necessary.		
5.	Places basin on a disposable absorbent pad at a comfortable position for the client. Immerses body part in water, padding the edge of the basin as necessary. Covers client for extra warmth if needed.		
6.	Checks water temperature every 5 minutes, adding hot water as needed.		
7.	Observes area for discoloration and discontinues soak if the client complains of pain or discomfort.		
8.	Soaks for 15–20 minutes or as ordered in the care plan.		
9.	Removes basin or helps client out of the tub. Dries the client.		
10.	Drains tub or empties basin in toilet. Rinses, cleans, and stores basin and other supplies. Puts laundry in hamper.		
11.	Washes hands.		
12.	Documents time, length, and site of procedure and any observations. Reports client's response and observations about skin.		

Date Reviewed ______ Instructor Signature ______

Date Performed ______ Instructor Signature ______

Using a hot-water bottle

		yes	no
1.	Washes hands.		
2.	Explains procedure to client, speaking clearly, slowly, and directly. Maintains face-to-face contact whenever possible.		
3.	Provides privacy.		
4.	Fills bottle halfway with warm water, presses out excess air, and seals bottle.		
5.	Dries the bottle and checks for leaks. Covers bottle with cloth or towel.		
6.	Applies bottle to the area. Checks skin every 5 minutes for discoloration or pain. Adds cold water to bottle if skin is red or client complains of pain.		
7.	Removes bottle after 20 minutes or as ordered in the care plan.		
8.	Empties bottle and washes and stores supplies.		
9.	Washes hands.		
10.	Documents time, length, and site of procedure, and any observations.		

Date Reviewed ______ Instructor Signature ______

Date Performed ______ Instructor Signature ______

Assisting with a sitz bath

		yes	no
1.	Washes hands.		
2.	Explains procedure to client, speaking clearly, slowly, and directly. Maintains face-to-face contact whenever possible.		
3.	Provides privacy.		
4.	Puts on gloves.		

Name: ____________________

		yes	no
5.	Fills sitz bath 2/3 full with warm water. Places sitz bath on toilet seat and checks water temperature.		
6.	Helps client undress and sit on sitz bath.		
7.	If leaving the room, checks on client every 5 minutes for weakness or dizziness. Stays with client who is unsteady.		
8.	Assists client off sitz bath after 20 minutes. Provides towels and helps with dressing as needed.		
9.	Cleans and stores supplies. Puts laundry in hamper.		
10.	Removes and discards gloves. Washes hands.		
11.	Documents procedure, including the time started and ended, the client's response, and the water temperature.		

Date Reviewed ____________ Instructor Signature ____________

Date Performed ____________ Instructor Signature ____________

Applying an ice pack

		yes	no
1.	Washes hands.		
2.	Explains procedure to client, speaking clearly, slowly, and directly. Maintains face-to-face contact whenever possible.		
3.	Provides privacy.		
4.	Fills plastic bag 1/2 to 2/3 full with ice and removes excess air. Covers bag with towel.		
5.	Applies bag to the area as ordered. Uses another towel to cover bag if it is too cold.		
6.	Notes the time and checks the area after 5 minutes for blisters or discolored skin. Stops treatment if client complains of numbness or pain.		
7.	Removes ice after 20 minutes or as ordered in the care plan. Returns ice bag to freezer. Puts laundry in hamper.		
8.	Washes hands.		
9.	Documents the time, length, and site of procedure. Reports the client's response and any observations about the skin.		

Date Reviewed ____________ Instructor Signature ____________

Date Performed ____________ Instructor Signature ____________

Changing a dry dressing using nonsterile technique

		yes	no
1.	Washes hands.		
2.	Explains procedure to client, speaking clearly, slowly, and directly. Maintains face-to-face contact whenever possible.		
3.	Provides privacy.		
4.	Places supplies on a clean bed protector or paper towel within reach. Opens gauze package without touching the gauze.		
5.	Puts on gloves.		
6.	Removes soiled dressing gently, observing dressing for odor or drainage. Notes color and size of the wound. Discards used dressing in the plastic bag.		
7.	Removes and discards gloves in the plastic bag. Washes hands.		
8.	Puts on clean gloves.		
9.	Applies clean gauze to wound. Tapes gauze in place, securing firmly.		

Name: ______________________

10.	Discards supplies.		
11.	Removes and discards gloves. Washes hands.		
12.	Documents procedure and any observations.		
	Date Reviewed / Instructor Signature		
	Date Performed / Instructor Signature		

Applying knee-high compression stockings

		yes	no
1.	Washes hands.		
2.	Explains procedure to client, speaking clearly, slowly, and directly. Maintains face-to-face contact whenever possible.		
3.	Provides privacy.		
4.	With client lying down in supine position, removes socks, shoes, or slippers, and exposes one leg.		
5.	Turns stocking inside out at least to heel area.		
6.	Gently places the foot of the stocking over toes, foot, and heel. Makes sure heel is in right place.		
7.	Gently pulls top of stocking over foot, heel, and leg.		
8.	Makes sure that there are no twists or wrinkles in the stocking after it is applied. Makes sure heel of stocking is over heel of foot.		
9.	Repeats for the other leg.		
10.	Washes hands.		
11.	Documents procedure and any observations.		
	Date Reviewed / Instructor Signature		
	Date Performed / Instructor Signature		

Caring for an ostomy

		yes	no
1.	Washes hands.		
2.	Explains procedure to client, speaking clearly, slowly, and directly. Maintains face-to-face contact whenever possible.		
3.	Provides privacy.		
4.	Adjusts bed to a safe working level. Locks bed wheels.		
5.	Puts on gloves.		
6.	Places bed protector under client. Covers client with a bath blanket and only exposes the ostomy site.		
7.	Removes ostomy pouch carefully and places in plastic bag. Notes color, odor, consistency, and amount of stool in the pouch.		
8.	Wipes area around the stoma with disposable wipes for ostomy care. Discards wipes in plastic bag.		
9.	Washes area around the stoma using a washcloth and warm soapy water. Moves in one direction, away from the stoma. Pats dry with another towel.		
10.	Places the clean ostomy pouch on client, following instructions. Seals securely. Makes sure the bottom of the pouch is clamped.		
11.	Removes disposable bed protector and discards. Discards plastic bag and places soiled linens in proper containers.		
12.	Removes and discards gloves. Washes hands.		
13.	Returns bed to lowest position.		

Name: ______________________

14.	Documents procedure and any observations.		
Date Reviewed	Instructor Signature		
Date Performed	Instructor Signature		

15
Medications and Technology in Home Care

Assisting in changing clothes for a client who has an IV

		yes	no
1.	Washes hands.		
2.	Explains procedure to client, speaking clearly, slowly, and directly. Maintains face-to-face contact whenever possible.		
3.	Provides privacy.		
4.	Adjusts bed to lowest position. Locks bed wheels. Helps client to sitting position with feet flat on the floor. Lets client sit for a few minutes.		
5.	Helps client remove the arm without the IV from the clothing.		
6.	Helps client gather clothing on arm with IV site, lifts clothing over IV site, and moves it up the tubing toward the IV bag.		
7.	Lifts IV bag off the pole, keeping it higher than the IV site, slides clothing over IV bag, and replaces IV bag on the pole.		
8.	Sets used clothing aside and gathers the sleeve of the clean clothing.		
9.	Lifts IV bag off the pole again, keeping it higher than the IV site, slides clean clothing over IV bag, and replaces IV bag on the pole.		
10.	Moves clean clothing over tubing and IV site and onto the client's arm.		
11.	Assists client with putting other arm into clothing.		
12.	Observes the IV for 1 minute to make sure that it is dripping properly. Checks the tubing and dressing for proper placement.		
13.	Assists client with changing the rest of her clothing.		
14.	Leaves bed in lowest position. Places soiled laundry in laundry hamper.		
15.	Washes hands.		
16.	Documents procedure and any observations.		
Date Reviewed	Instructor Signature		
Date Performed	Instructor Signature		

16
Rehabilitation and Restorative Care

Assisting with passive range of motion exercises

		yes	no
1.	Washes hands.		
2.	Explains procedure to client, speaking clearly, slowly, and directly. Maintains face-to-face contact whenever possible.		
3.	Provides privacy.		
4.	Adjusts bed to a safe working level. Locks bed wheels.		
5.	Positions client in supine position. Repeats each exercise at least 3 times.		

Name: ___________________________

	Shoulder: Performs the following movements properly, supporting the client's arm at the elbow and wrist by placing one hand under the elbow and the other hand under the wrist:		
a.	Extension		
b.	Flexion		
c.	Abduction		
d.	Adduction		
	Elbow: Performs the following movements properly, holding the wrist with one hand and holding the elbow with the other:		
a.	Flexion		
b.	Extension		
c.	Pronation		
d.	Supination		
	Wrist: Performs the following movements properly, holding the wrist with one hand and using the fingers of the other hand to help the joint through the motions:		
a.	Flexion		
b.	Dorsiflexion		
c.	Radial flexion		
d.	Ulnar flexion		
	Thumb: Performs the following movements properly:		
a.	Abduction		
b.	Adduction		
c.	Opposition		
d.	Flexion		
e.	Extension		
	Fingers: Performs the following movements properly:		
a.	Flexion		
b.	Extension		
c.	Abduction		
d.	Adduction		
	Hip: Performs the following movements properly, placing one hand under the knee and one under the ankle:		
a.	Abduction		
b.	Adduction		
c.	Internal rotation		
d.	External rotation		
	Knees: Performs the following movements properly, placing one hand under the knee and one under the ankle:		
a.	Flexion		
b.	Extension		
	Ankles: Performs the following movements while properly supporting the foot and ankle:		
a.	Dorsiflexion		
b.	Plantar flexion		
c.	Supination		
d.	Pronation		
	Toes: Performs the following movements properly:		
a.	Flexion		
b.	Extension		
c.	Abduction		
6.	***When all exercises are completed:*** Returns client to comfortable position and covers as appropriate. Returns bed to its lowest position.		
7.	Washes hands.		

Name: ____________________

8.	Documents procedure. Notes any decrease in range of motion or any pain experienced by the client. Notifies supervisor if increased stiffness or physical resistance is noted.		

Date Reviewed ______ Instructor Signature ______

Date Performed ______ Instructor Signature ______

Assisting with deep breathing exercises

		yes	no
1.	Washes hands.		
2.	Explains procedure to client, speaking clearly, slowly, and directly. Maintains face-to-face contact whenever possible.		
3.	Provides privacy.		
4.	Puts on gown, mask, and goggles as indicated (using N95 if client has or may have tuberculosis).		
5.	Puts on gloves.		
6.	Has client breathe in slowly and steadily while sitting up.		
7.	Has client exhale completely.		
8.	Repeats exercise 5 to 10 times.		
9.	Offers tissues or emesis basin as necessary.		
10.	Disposes of tissues and cleans and stores basin.		
11.	Removes gloves, goggles, gown, and mask.		
12.	Washes hands.		
13.	Puts on new gloves.		
14.	Provides mouth care.		
15.	Removes and discards gloves. Washes hands.		
16.	Documents procedure and any observations.		

Date Reviewed ______ Instructor Signature ______

Date Performed ______ Instructor Signature ______

19
New Mothers, Infants, and Children

Picking up and holding a baby

		yes	no
1.	Washes hands.		
2.	Supports the head at all times when lifting or holding a baby. With the other hand, supports the baby's back and bottom.		
3.	Performs cradle hold properly.		
4.	Performs football hold properly.		
5.	Performs upright hold properly.		

Date Reviewed ______ Instructor Signature ______

Date Performed ______ Instructor Signature ______

Sterilizing bottles

		yes	no
1.	Washes hands.		
2.	Boils water and puts equipment in, ensuring it is all submerged.		
3.	Reboils water for 5 minutes.		
4.	Removes equipment and discards water. Stores when dry.		

Date Reviewed ______ Instructor Signature ______

Date Performed ______ Instructor Signature ______

Assisting with bottle-feeding			
		yes	no
1.	Washes hands.		
2.	Prepares bottle.		
3.	Sits and holds baby properly.		
4.	Inserts bottle nipple, and ensures that baby's head is higher than body.		
5.	Talks or sings to baby during feeding.		
6.	Burps baby, changes diaper, and puts baby down.		
7.	Washes hands.		
8.	Documents procedure and any observations.		
9.	Washes and sterilizes bottle, nipple, and ring.		
Date Reviewed	Instructor Signature		
Date Performed	Instructor Signature		

Burping a baby			
		yes	no
1.	Washes hands.		
2.	Picks up baby, using either of the two safe positions.		
3.	Pats back gently until baby burps.		
4.	Returns baby to a safe place.		
Date Reviewed	Instructor Signature		
Date Performed	Instructor Signature		

Giving an infant a sponge bath			
		yes	no
1.	Washes hands.		
2.	Puts on gloves.		
3.	Gathers supplies. Fills basin and tests water temperature.		
4.	Holds baby in football hold and washes eyes, then rest of face, using no soap.		
5.	Holds baby in football hold and washes hair.		
6.	Lays baby down, keeping one hand on baby.		
7.	Undresses upper body and washes it. Dries and covers the baby.		
8.	Undresses lower body and washes and dries it.		
9.	Washes perineal area properly.		
10.	Washes bottom and dries completely.		
11.	Applies lotion, keeping baby covered.		
12.	Diapers and dresses baby. Returns baby to a safe place.		
13.	Discards water, puts towels in the laundry, cleans supplies, and discards gloves.		
14.	Washes hands.		
15.	Documents procedure and any observations.		
Date Reviewed	Instructor Signature		
Date Performed	Instructor Signature		

Giving an infant a tub bath			
		yes	no
1.	Washes hands.		
2.	Puts on gloves.		
3.	Gathers supplies. Fills basin and tests water temperature.		
4.	Holds baby in football hold and washes eyes, then rest of face, using no soap.		

Name: ______________________

5.	Holds baby in football hold and washes hair.		
6.	Lays baby down, undresses, and immerses baby in basin, keeping head above water.		
7.	Uses washcloth to wash from neck down.		
8.	Removes baby from bath and covers immediately.		
9.	Applies lotion, keeping baby covered as much as possible.		
10.	Diapers and dresses baby. Returns baby to a safe place.		
11.	Discards water, puts towels in the laundry, cleans supplies, and discards gloves.		
12.	Washes hands.		
13.	Documents procedure and any observations.		

Date Reviewed ____________ Instructor Signature ____________

Date Performed ____________ Instructor Signature ____________

Changing cloth or disposable diapers

		yes	no
1.	Washes hands.		
2.	Puts on gloves.		
3.	Undresses baby and removes diaper, keeping one hand on the baby at all times.		
4.	Cleans perineal area.		
5.	Applies ointment as necessary and allows air to circulate.		
6.	Applies cloth or disposable diaper properly.		
7.	Dresses baby and returns to a safe place.		
8.	Disposes of diaper properly.		
9.	Removes and discards gloves. Washes hands.		
10.	Cleans area and stores supplies.		

11.	Washes hands again.		
12.	Documents procedure and any observations.		

Date Reviewed ____________ Instructor Signature ____________

Date Performed ____________ Instructor Signature ____________

Measuring and recording a baby's weight

		yes	no
1.	Washes hands.		
2.	Places infant scale on firm surface. Places clean paper on scale and starts with scale at 0.		
3.	Undresses baby. Places baby on scale, keeping one hand on baby at all times.		
4.	Reads and remembers weight.		
5.	Removes baby and dresses him. Returns to a safe place.		
6.	Washes hands.		
7.	Documents procedure and any observations.		

Date Reviewed ____________ Instructor Signature ____________

Date Performed ____________ Instructor Signature ____________

Measuring and recording a baby's length

		yes	no
1.	Washes hands.		
2.	Prepares firm surface with clean sheet of paper with inch markings.		
3.	Places baby on surface, keeping one hand on baby at all times.		
4.	Places baby's head at beginning of measured marks. Straightens one knee and makes a mark on the paper at baby's heel.		
5.	Determines and remembers length.		

Name: ______________________

6.	Removes baby and returns to a safe position.		
7.	Washes hands.		
8.	Documents procedure and any observations.		
1.	***When paper with inch markings is not available:*** Washes hands.		
2.	Prepares firm surface with plain sheet of paper longer than the baby.		
3.	Places baby on surface, keeping one hand on baby at all times.		
4.	Makes pencil mark on the paper at top of baby's head. Straightens one knee and makes a mark on the paper at baby's heel. Removes baby and returns to a safe place.		
5.	Measures distance between marks with tape measure. Remembers length.		
6.	Washes hands.		
7.	Documents procedure and any observations.		

Date Reviewed ____________ Instructor Signature ____________

Date Performed ____________ Instructor Signature ____________

Measuring and recording an infant's axillary, tympanic, or temporal artery temperature

		yes	no
1.	Washes hands.		
2.	Prepares thermometer.		
3.	***For axillary temperature:*** Undresses baby on one side and lays baby down. Places tip of thermometer under the arm. Keeps thermometer in place for 3 to 5 minutes or until signal sounds.		
	For tympanic temperature: Lays baby on her side. Gently pulls outside of the ear toward back of head. Inserts thermometer tip into ear and presses button. Holds until thermometer blinks or beeps.		
	For temporal artery temperature: Turns on thermometer and places it flat on baby's forehead. Presses and holds scan button and sweeps thermometer across the forehead, keeping contact with the baby's skin. Releases scan button.		
4.	Removes thermometer and reads temperature, keeping one hand on baby. Dresses baby and returns to a safe place.		
5.	Cleans and stores thermometer and supplies.		
6.	Washes hands.		
7.	Documents temperature.		

Date Reviewed ____________ Instructor Signature ____________

Date Performed ____________ Instructor Signature ____________

21
Clean, Safe, and Healthy Environments

Cleaning a bathroom

		yes	no
1.	Puts on gloves.		
2.	Wipes all surfaces with disinfectant and rag or wipe.		
3.	Cleans bathtub, shower, and sink, using a different rag.		
4.	Wipes toilet bowl, using a different rag.		
5.	Scrubs inside of toilet bowl with brush and flushes toilet.		

Name: ______________________

		yes	no
6.	Vacuums or sweeps, then washes, floor.		
7.	Cleans mirror and all glass.		
8.	Places soiled rags in laundry and disposes of waste.		
9.	Stores supplies.		
10.	Removes and discards gloves. Washes hands.		
11.	Documents procedure and any observations.		

Date Reviewed ____________ Instructor Signature ____________

Date Performed ____________ Instructor Signature ____________

Doing the laundry

		yes	no
1.	Sorts clothes carefully, checking pockets and garments.		
2.	Pretreats clothes as necessary.		
3.	Uses correct temperature, laundry products, and washing cycle.		
4.	Dries clothes.		
5.	Hand washes as necessary.		
6.	Folds and hangs clean laundry. Stores clothes.		

Date Reviewed ____________ Instructor Signature ____________

Date Performed ____________ Instructor Signature ____________

Making an occupied bed

		yes	no
1.	Washes hands.		
2.	Explains procedure to client, speaking clearly, slowly, and directly. Maintains face-to-face contact whenever possible.		
3.	Provides privacy.		
4.	Places clean linen on clean surface within reach.		
5.	Adjusts bed to a safe working level. Locks bed wheels.		
6.	Puts on gloves.		
7.	Loosens top linen from working side and covers client. Removes top sheet.		
8.	Raises side rail on far side of bed. Goes to other side and turns client onto her side, toward raised rail.		
9.	Loosens bottom soiled linen, mattress pad, and protector on working side.		
10.	Rolls bottom soiled linen toward client, tucking it snugly against the client's back.		
11.	Places and tucks in clean bottom linen, finishing with no wrinkles. Makes hospital corners if necessary.		
12.	Smoothes bottom sheet out toward the client. Rolls extra material toward client and tucks it under client's body.		
13.	Places disposable absorbent pad if using and centers it. Smoothes it out toward client and tucks it under client's body.		
14.	Places draw sheet if using. Smoothes and tucks as with other bedding.		
15.	Raises side rail on working side and goes to other side of bed and lowers that rail. Assists client to turn onto clean bottom sheet, toward the raised rail.		
16.	Loosens soiled linen. Rolls linen from head to the foot of bed, avoiding contact with skin or clothes. Places it in a laundry hamper or basket.		

Name: ______________________

		yes	no
17.	Pulls and tucks in clean bottom linen just like other side, finishing with bottom sheet free of wrinkles. Makes hospital corners if necessary.		
18.	Asks client to turn onto her back, keeping client covered. Raises side rail nearest self.		
19.	Unfolds top sheet and places it over client. Slips blanket or old sheet out from underneath. Puts it in the laundry hamper.		
20.	Places a blanket over the top sheet, matching the top edges. Tucks bottom edges of top sheet and blanket under mattress, making square corners on each side. Loosens top linens over client's feet. Folds top sheet over the blanket about 6 inches.		
21.	Removes pillow and pillowcase. Places pillowcase in the laundry hamper. Removes and discards gloves. Washes hands.		
22.	Places clean pillowcases on pillows. Places them under client's head.		
23.	Returns bed to lowest position. Leaves side rails in ordered position. Carries laundry hamper to laundry area.		
24.	Washes hands.		
25.	Documents procedure and any observations.		

Date Reviewed ____________ Instructor Signature ____________

Date Performed ____________ Instructor Signature ____________

Making an unoccupied bed

		yes	no
1.	Washes hands.		
2.	Places clean linen on clean surface within reach.		
3.	Adjusts bed to a safe working level. Locks bed wheels.		
4.	Puts on gloves.		
5.	Loosens soiled linen and rolls it from head to foot of bed. Avoids contact with skin or clothes. Places it in a hamper or basket. Removes pillows and pillowcases and places pillowcases in hamper.		
6.	Removes and discards gloves. Washes hands.		
7.	Remakes bed, spreading mattress pad and bottom sheet, tucking under. Makes hospital corners. Puts on disposable absorbent pad and draw sheet, smoothes, and tucks under sides of bed.		
8.	Places top sheet and blanket, centering them. Tucks under end of bed and makes hospital corners. Folds down top sheet over the blanket about 6 inches.		
9.	Puts on clean pillowcases. Replaces pillows.		
10.	Returns bed to its lowest position. Carries laundry hamper to laundry area.		
11.	Washes hands.		
12.	Documents procedure and any observations.		

Date Reviewed ____________ Instructor Signature ____________

Date Performed ____________ Instructor Signature ____________

Name: ______________________

22
Clients' Nutritional Needs

Assisting a client with eating

		yes	no
1.	Washes hands.		
2.	Explains procedure to client, speaking clearly, slowly, and directly. Maintains face-to-face contact whenever possible.		
3.	Provides privacy.		
4.	Positions client in upright sitting position. Adjusts bed height to be sitting at client's eye level. Locks bed wheels.		
5.	Places food and drink where they can be easily seen by the client.		
6.	Helps client to wash hands. Helps client to put on clothing protector if desired.		
7.	Sits facing client at client's eye level on stronger side.		
8.	Tells the client what foods are on the plate. Asks what she would like to eat first. Checks temperature of food. Offers food in bite-sized pieces and alternates types of food offered. Makes sure client's mouth is empty before offering the next bite of food or sip of drink.		
9.	Offers drinks throughout the meal. Talks throughout the meal.		
10.	Wipes client's mouth and hands as necessary.		
11.	Removes clothing protector if used. Removes tray or dishes.		
12.	Assists client to a comfortable position, keeping client upright for at least 30 minutes. Returns bed to lowest position.		
13.	Washes hands.		
14.	Documents procedure (including client's intake if required) and any observations.		

Date Reviewed	Instructor Signature
Date Performed	Instructor Signature